F I T N E S S
S T R E T C H I N G

In memory of Gwendolyn Stewart Jerome Luer
1907–1985

ACKNOWLEDGMENTS

This book grew out of conversations with several talented and generous individuals, most of whom helped guide my subsequent research. I owe a large debt of gratitude to Dr. Theodore J. Becker, Stephen A. Black, Dr. David L. Costill, Dr. Sandra Curwin, Fred Dalby, Dr. Richard H. Dominguez, Dr. E. C. Frederick, Dr. Dennis Golden, Marijeanne Liederbach, Dr. Alan Magid, Michael Marino, Dr. Thomas A. McMahon, Dr. James Nicholas, Dr. Roy J. Shephard, Mary C. Staggs, and Dr. William D. Stanish. I would especially like to thank Dr. R. Keith McCormick and family and staff, and my wife, Chris, who not only helped with research but were of invaluable assistance in shaping the final manuscript, and Hans Teensma, who guided the illustrations through to completion.

CONTENTS

AUTHOR'S NOTE

The information contained in this book is intended to complement, not substitute for, the advice of your own physician, with whom you should always consult before starting any medical or physical regime. The exercises described in this book are very beneficial but may not be recommended for people with special medical problems. Always ask your doctor about any specific questions or problems you may have.

INTRODUCTION

Exercise is work, but it's also pleasure, and pleasure is the part that keeps us at it. Traditional exercise programs, with their no pain, no gain emphasis on progressive overload, often work against themselves. They teach us that hard effort can be pleasurable, and we learn the lesson too well, coming to love our daily exertions too dearly. We find ourselves bringing the same obsessive energies to exercise that we used to reserve for careers, crusades, love affairs, and other great passions. The results range from morning-after soreness to severe orthopedic problems. Overuse injuries are our pesky new plague.

"Overuse" means an unfitting level of use. To fit the work accurately to the needs of the body may require that we take a little off our level of effort, that we ease up on our determination always to do a bit more. To serious athletes and other die-hard exercisers this may sound subversive, but it represents a great sea-change in current athletic thinking. If your recreational history has been subject to the occasional interruption, or has simply been insufficiently rewarding, the time may have come to acquire a little more tolerance and flexibility in your attitudes toward athletic effort.

Flexibility, it turns out, is the significant metaphor. Serious athletes—the ones who last for very long, anyway—eventually come to understand that the single physical asset most critical to continued and successful hard use of the human body isn't strength or speed or endurance, but suppleness. Suppleness—loose and easy flexibility—is the quality that defends against the harshness of our athletic experience; it slows the abruptness with which we approach our physical limits; it softens the blows. It is the source of our elasticity, the spring-loading in the biomechanics of athletics. Suppleness is the resilience of specific body tissues, but it is also the resilience of our larger systems, the capacity to adjust to a wide range of demands, athletic or otherwise. Suppleness of tissue contributes to suppleness of everything else; there is a direct physiological link between these two kinds of resilience. This book is about maintenance of that link.

One of the tools for its maintenance is stretching. Among serious athletes and their trainers, stretching has become almost universally accepted as the best technique for warming up and cooling down, as preparation for action and as therapy for its excesses. Yet stretching remains controversial, because it is poorly understood even by its greatest supporters. There has been a fundamental omission in the way the world of athletics has perceived stretching. One aim of this book is to correct that omission, and clear up the controversies and mysteries that surround the simple act. Another aim is to present a different way to stretch.

The soft tissue of the musculoskeletal system—principally the muscle and the connective tissue—responds to overuse by shrinking and tightening. Its response to *under*use, mysteriously, is much the same. We know perfectly well that injury causes "stiffness" (whatever that is), that inactivity causes stiffness, that aging causes stiffness. But we have it backward: stiffness is the cause, not the result. You don't lose suppleness because you get old or out of shape, you get old or out of shape—or injured— because you've lost suppleness. Maintaining full physical effectiveness is a matter of balancing levels of use to retain suppleness. That's what *Staying Supple* is all about.

Part I of this book is concerned with how one stays supple, Part II with the physiology of suppleness, and Part III with its loss. On the assumption that the better you understand something the better you can apply it, there's a fair amount of technical material in the following pages. Some ideas are introduced early, and their physiological rationale saved for later, which may appear repetitious. My apologies for that: it's a complex subject, and every part of it can't come first. A glossary follows the text, for quick reference. Chapters 6 and 7 in particular are intended for those who are fascinated by the particle and detail of physiological matters; less technical-minded readers may want to skip them. If you are eager to get started, you might want to read chapter 4 first—preferably while lying on a stretching mat—and enjoy yourself. I like to think that the enjoyment will increase if you then go back and read the rest.

Staying Supple is, in other words, a how-to book, but of a different kind, I hope. How-to books drive me crazy. I have a love-hate relationship with them, buying them by the armfuls, squirming with frustration when I read them. Exercise how-to books are dependably the worst, telling you precisely how many times to do things and exactly what position you are to assume, and otherwise ignoring the astonishing physical variety of our species—on the assumption, I suppose, that we are too busy or too passive to care how things really work. The gospel of the how-to business seems to be that the reader doesn't want anything to think about, but only to be promised a great deal and then led, step by mechanical step, through a rigid program. If you're that reader, chapter 4 is about as close as this book will come to meeting your needs. What is presented here is not yet another fitness program, but a way of understanding how your musculoskeletal system prefers to work, and of putting that understanding to effective use. A few specific movements are presented, mostly to stimulate your imagination. They are intended only as starting places: you'll end up creating your own program to fit your body and its needs.

Although there is much talk of scientific matters in these pages, this is an experiential rather than a scientific book. Science, with its need for numbers and objective verification, isn't very good at examining the softer qualities, and studies in this area have not been as productive as the popular press would lead us to believe. I have surveyed the available science, but I've also relied on my experience and that of others. Much of the evidence I've relied on is what science calls anecdotal.

In that sense I suppose what follows is Eastern, rather than Western, in viewpoint. Western science distrusts subjective experience; Eastern science doesn't. In fact, Eastern science tends not to trust any phenomenon that can't be experienced directly; anything else is only theory. There's no intention here of being antiscience or anti-Western, but when you're working with your own body—your own pain and pleasure receptors—the Eastern approach has much to recommend it.

But don't trust my experience, trust your own. Check these matters out for yourself. This book is about pleasure—the pleasure of using a body that has full natural resilience and flexibility, and the equal pleasure to be gained from the very process of maintaining that suppleness. Approach it with that in mind, and the benefits—the improvements to the physical plant that result—are pure bonus.

PART I

STAYING

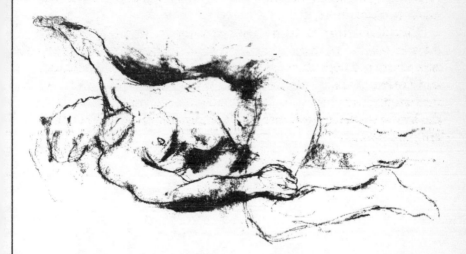

SUPPLE

ONE

SPECIFICITY AND THE ONE-PIECE BODY

The human body comes in one flexible piece. If you don't treat it that way, you're asking for trouble. Unfortunately, modern athletic practice is based almost entirely on the principle of specificity, and the first casualty of the specific approach is our understanding of the body as a one-piece unit.

Specificity means that the gains from training are limited to those parts of the body and those physiological systems that are being worked. This seems obvious, but it's surprising how often, in the frustrating struggle to improve performance, we forget it. It means that training trains only the specific systems, the specific muscles and nerves and biochemical transactions, that you are actually using. Training for marathons won't condition you for a Sunday afternoon game of touch football—or even, in the fine-grained approach of the serious athlete, for running 10-K races. Lifting weights trains the muscles only for lifting weights, not for tennis or skiing.

Moreover, specificity decrees that weightlifting trains only the specific muscles used, and trains them only for lifting weights through the specific motions you practice, at the speed you practice them. Claims of aerobic conditioning from continuous, fast-paced weight-machine work, for instance, have not proved out. "Cross-training," the attempt to improve performance in one athletic discipline by training for another, is a recent fad; in practice, cross-training simply reduces the rate of gain—when it doesn't actually reduce outright performance—in both disciplines. It takes training time and energy away from the specific areas that will contribute to higher performance. The triathlon was invented to circumvent this narrow-gauge approach, but it turns out that triathlon winners are those who do the most training in the three specific disciplines of the event. Specificity is a fact of athletic life.

Once we began looking to science to improve athletic performance, the specific approach was inevitable. The business of science is measurement, and scientists can't measure what they can't isolate. Experiments are worthless unless controls can be set up so that a single variable can be traced. Given this requirement, sports science could hardly come up with anything but specificity as the key to maximum athletic improvement. So modern athletics becomes ever more reductionist, in search of the critical factors that make one athletic effort more successful than the next.

Specificity works. The specific approach to training is responsible for the explosion of world records and other spectacular athletic performances in recent years. Athletic technicians are increasingly able to pinpoint and guide improvement of the precise physical systems necessary to achieve specific athletic goals. Computers analyze everything from the sequence of muscle contractions in the shot put to the blood chemistry of middle-distance swimmers; training techniques capitalize on the data. Specificity is also responsible for a phenomenal improvement in the reduction and rehabilitation of injuries. As we've learned more about which parts of the anatomy are involved in which motions—about which tissues support which loads—we've been able to direct the strengthening and healing of those elements much more accurately.

But there's one category of athletic injuries that is caused *by* specificity in athletic training, and it has become epidemic in recent years. These are the injuries of overuse; they occur when some aspect of the athletic plant simply wears out. Zeroing in on an athletic task necessarily means loading a narrower set of physical systems. The load is no longer shared, but is brought to bear on ever smaller areas; the points of wear become more acute. The line between training and overtraining is narrowed. Tipping the balance from improvement into breakdown becomes much harder to avoid. Something is much more likely to give.

When that happens, a larger principle than specificity is at work: it is the principle that says that the body comes in one flexible piece. It works better, it improves more, it lasts longer when you use it that way.

Scientists acknowledge this one-piece, interlocking nature of the body, despite their difficulty in figuring out how to work with it. We think of aerobic exercise, for instance, as training that starts with the heart, but there's a view that it really starts by training skeletal muscle. Dr. George Sheehan, the cardiologist and running guru, mischievously suggests that running trains only the legs—which then drag everything else along with them. Leg muscles grow more efficient at producing energy and removing wastes, which means that they can process more blood (which trains the heart muscle) and more oxygen (which trains the lungs), and so on throughout the cardiovascular system. New bone material is laid down, tendons strengthened, nerve pathways reinforced. The interconnectedness of these systems makes the designation of any starting point purely arbitrary. This is the one-piece view of athletic physiology, which would seem to make a mockery of specificity.

The one-piece view, however, is a relatively inefficient approach to preparation for the highest levels of athletic competition. There will always be specific strengths and weaknesses that athletes want to address, and they will use specific training methods to address them. Specificity isn't going to go away. If the athletic goal is a single off-scale performance, with no concern for the consequences, specificity is the best approach science can come up with for achieving it. This is precisely how many extremely talented athletes approach their tasks. They tend to have great successes—and brief careers. The costs of the specific approach are, too often, unacceptably high.

If the athletic effort is launched from a supple physiological base, however, not only can those high costs be reduced, but even the off-scale performances can be improved. The elite-level athletes who last, who continue to perform well over extended careers, come to understand this well enough. Nonelites can benefit from the same lesson. For most of us, the goal is not a single record-breaking performance but a lifetime of pleasurable physical activity. For that, you really do need a supple body. Specificity won't give you one.

THE FOURTH VARIABLE

Specificity brings a reductionist view to the athletic process. That view proposes that speed, strength, and endurance are the critical athletic attributes. Analysts assure us that, all else being equal, the faster athlete will win—in any sport, any physical contest. Speed is so critical that today's scouts attempt to reduce it to component parts, speaking of "foot speed" or "quickness" as somehow different from sheer speed. (As baseball pitchers began, a few years ago, to talk of "velocity.") Along with the conventional vital statistics of height, weight, and age, the pro's personnel file now contains an additional number: time for the 40-yard dash.

But, the same experts tell us, if all contending athletes are equal in speed, the stronger will prevail. And in the unlikely event that all are equally fast and equally strong, then obviously the winner will be the one who lasts longest, who can maintain the speed and continue to exert the force longer than the others. Endurance will provide the final measure.

All else is never equal, of course, in athletics or anything else. Athletic performance is a blend of attributes; the winner isn't necessarily the fastest or the strongest, but the one who can apply speed at the proper moment, bring force to bear in the proper place. What wins is the *appropriate* use of physical and mental resources. The experts know this, but can't find a way to measure it. They're stuck with measuring what they can, reporting what they can get their numbers on—straight-line force, obvious speed, time-to-failure. With luck, something will translate.

Specificity's emphasis on speed, strength, and endurance means that insufficient attention is paid to the fourth physical attribute, the one that literally as well as figuratively ties the other three together, which is suppleness: flexibility. Working to maintain and improve suppleness is in a sense the only cross-training that really works; it is training of the ground substance through which all effort is made, the athletic tissue itself. It is specific to the degree that its target is tissue, that it focuses on improving the texture, quality, and health *of* tissue, but it is nonspecific in that it is aimed at no specific motion, no sport, no skill; it is aimed at improving every athletic response. It is the athlete's ultimate base, the base upon which you build the endurance, strength, and speed of the conventional wisdom.

Unfortunately, we know a great deal more about training for speed, strength, and endurance than we do about training for suppleness. Suppleness has a way of eluding the fixed principles of the scientific method. We're not even sure what we're talking about. People in sports sometimes use the term *flexible* to mean joints that are anatomically loose or sloppy, and sometimes they use it to refer to an arc of skeletal motion unhampered by tight muscles or tendons. The first usage blames hard tissue for limitations on motion; the second blames soft tissue. Both are attempts to describe athletic flexibility more simply and clearly—more scientifically—but they only muddy the picture.

The broader dictionary definition, applied not just to the athletic body but to any substance, is more useful. Both "flexible" and "supple," says *Webster's*, describe the ability to bend or fold easily, "without creases, cracks, breaks, or other injuries." For an athletic body, that ought to be the minimum starting point.

Definitions are abstractions; they become clearer when you flesh them out with pictures from real life. Watch experienced athletes. They don't warm up, they "get loose." They stir slowly into motion, sometimes making the moves of their particular sport but sometimes not—fiddling around with their athletic tools, in effect, until they reach a tension-free kind of confidence that they're ready for real effort: "I'm loose, coach, send me in."

They don't pursue warmth, they pursue bounciness, elasticity, fluidity. (Warmth is a by-product.) The goal is to get the soft tissue restored to its best working length, the joints lubricated, the synapses charged. Watch the pitcher warming up on the mound and the batter swinging away in the on-deck circle; both are rehearsing neural pathways, reminding nerves, muscles, and tendons just how to do the next demanding thing. Looseness is also a state of mind, much admired: tight minds make tight muscles, which make not only injuries but tentative movements, turnovers, booted plays. Tight minds make bad athletes.

Looseness *is* suppleness: it is flexibility in the conventional sense, but with the addition of quick resilience, a springy capacity to recover quickly. It is easy elasticity plus quick recoil or rebound. It is pure *liveliness;* it comes from healthy tissue, ready for action. Such suppleness is clearly a kind of safety net, a shock absorption system for the body. That makes it seem a defensive quality, passive, vaguely negative. In fact it is an extremely positive quality, contributing directly and immediately to improved athletic performance.

I once asked Olympic gold-medalist Tim Daggett about flexibility in gymnastics, expecting him to talk about reduced injuries and about the contorted positions that gymnasts must achieve. Instead, he spoke of the active contribution flexibility makes to gymnastic performance. "If you're not flexible," he said, "you won't be strong, because you won't get a big motion started. If you don't have much range of motion, you won't have as much power." He was talking practical physics: the bigger the move, the longer the arc through which to apply force. (Work is force times distance, and power is work divided by time.)

The same principles apply in all sports, although their application may be subtler than in the acrobatic contortions of gymnastics. Running is perhaps the most elemental athletic movement of all, and would seem to demand minimal flexibility. More than one high-level runner is fond of pointing this out, making fun of the stretching antics of fellow runners. (There are world-class marathoners who can't touch their toes.) A supple body is required for running the hurdles, perhaps, and other such specialized forms of track sports, but how much flexibility do you actually need just to run down the road?

More than you might believe, if you want to run swiftly and efficiently—and comfortably—down that road. The less ankle flexibility you have, for example, the shorter the arc through which you will be able to apply driving force against the ground. With a briefer arc, you'll expend more energy to attain the same speed. (Extend your stride one inch and you gain 20 yards per mile.) Moreover, the normal running stride never pulls the hamstring out to its full length, so hamstrings tend to shorten with distance training (if you don't stretch). A shortened hamstring resists every lift of the knee, sapping energy and reducing efficiency.

Brant Tolsma, Ph.D., track coach at Campbell University, published these and other observations in *Running Times* ("Flexibility and Velocity," June 1982). In addition to the defensive, injury-preventive aspects of flexibility, Tolsma points out, there are two very positive reasons for runners to pursue flexibility: increased range of force application and decreased range of muscular resistance. "Increasing the range over which a force is applied will increase the time of application of the force, resulting in a higher velocity," says Tolsma: i.e., you go faster. Decreasing muscular resistance reduces energy expenditure, increasing endurance: i.e., you go faster *longer*.

Tolsma's is the specific approach, focusing on the detail of ankle joint and hamstring, and it is correct, of course. Tim Daggett, on the other hand—practicing athlete rather than scientist—is talking about the hard use of a one-piece body. He's correct too: on the high bar or the tumbling mat, range of motion is never determined by a single joint. How far back you can reach overhead is not determined solely by shoulder joints but also by the flexibility of spine and hips, by the state of stomach muscles, even by the sense of balance. Flexibility is maintained—mostly—on a joint-by-joint basis, but its usefulness, its application, is on a whole-body basis.

Dancers, divers, and gymnasts don't need to be sold on flexibility training, but athletes whose sports require less extreme body positions tend to be a little stubborn about accepting its role in proper athletic preparation. When they resist the idea, it's usually because they've never gone beyond speed, strength, and endurance in their thinking about the athletic equation. They see athletics too specifically. It's ironic. Athletics is about action. Every action has an equal and opposite reaction. Every ounce of force you generate acts on your body with just as much force as it acts on the external world. Suppleness is the shock absorber for that force.

Specificity asks you to prepare each part of yourself separately; suppleness says it's okay, even helpful, to apply your entire self to the problem—and it provides the means of holding yourself together while you do it. Specificity asks the athlete to see himself or herself as a collection of bits and pieces, a package of diverse capabilities somehow all to be brought to bear on the athletic problem. Suppleness reminds the athlete to stay whole: to *be* the solution to the athletic task.

Specificity isn't "wrong," and it does work. It is the fastest and easiest way to improve some aspects of performance. It can also, through overuse, take you out of the game.

TWO

STRETCHING

To stay supple you must maintain the health and resilience of your connective tissue and the muscle it contains. Regular stretching helps maintain that health and resilience. If you are an athlete or a regular exerciser, this advice probably isn't new to you, although you may have been asked to take it on faith. Nobody ever quite says what stretching is and does. I'd like to try to rectify that.

Stretching instructions used to speak only of muscle, but a wave of recent stretching information has changed the emphasis to the connective tissue. Both are correct, but it helps to keep in mind the connective tissue, more than muscle, when you stretch. If you think only of stretching muscle, you're not as likely to find stretching a satisfying and fruitful activity.

When you stretch, you place muscle and connective tissue under a lengthening tension. To stretch effectively you must relax the muscles while you're stretching them: the resistance to the stretch should come from the elasticity of the tissues, not from the contraction of the muscle. An ideal stretching program would regularly take all of the articulated segments of the body through their full range of motion, but that's asking a little much even from full-time athletes; most people settle for consistent, regular stretching of the muscles and tendons that work the major joints, or those that are hardest used.

The available evidence suggests that regular stretching enhances performance and reduces injuries. Stretching also speeds the recovery and reduces the soreness that results from the work. It helps resist the gradual shortening and tightening of tissue that otherwise sets in from both over- and underuse, reducing the discomfort and slowing the progressive loss of capacity that accompany this tightening. And stretching helps neurologically, keeping the proprioceptive system tuned, the muscles' tone and reactivity balanced, one's sense of personal dimension sharp and accurate.

Stretching accomplishes all these things mostly by restoring freshness. It is assumed to help straighten out the mechanical results of fatigue, physically reorganizing muscle and connective tissue fibers into their proper order—training them, in effect, to seek and maintain their optimum length. It also helps wash out the chemical residues of fatigue: the acids and other metabolic wastes that impair healing, slow the restoration of energy supplies, and hasten the mechanical shortening of tissue.

The mechanical refurbishment of muscle and connective tissue fibers from stretching is an accepted technique in orthopedic rehabilitation, although it is not easy to demonstrate in the laboratory. I don't know that the improvement in circulation from stretching has been measured either, but the mechanism to accomplish it is clear enough. Stretching works the one-way venous pumps in skeletal muscle, speeding the returning blood flow. Circulation of lymphatic fluids (which fight infection and remove wastes) and synovial fluids (which lubricate joint surfaces) are also surely stimulated, although the mechanisms for that are a little less direct. Of course, ordinary muscular contraction—exercise itself—boosts circulation in similar ways. But when muscular contractions are working the pumps, they're burning energy, and thus generating new wastes, at the same time. Stretching keeps on cleaning up when the factory is shut down. It also tidies things up before work starts—laying out the tools and supplies, so to speak, for ready access.

In addition, stretching seems to help quiet the neuromuscular noise that leaves muscle with those knots, spasms, and kernels of pain that you can't quite relax, that your best intentions can't reach. Physiology is strikingly vague about what these knots are and what causes them, but as surely as muscles contract in response to neural signals, they must fail to *de*contract because they're still getting some kind of residual signaling—"noise," in physics. (This signaling is produced in part by the irritation caused by waste products. Pain is one kind of noise.) Stretching should interrupt those unresolved contractions mechanically, helping restore normal function. This has not been proved, only demonstrated.

One explanation offered for the knots and spasms is *fibrosis*—abnormal formation of fibrous tissue, another poorly understood phenomenon. Injured muscle fibers have limited capacity to repair themselves; any large deficit is replaced by connective tissue. The smaller, microscopic tissue ruptures that are a natural product of hard use, called *microtrauma*, also must be healed. How much of that repair is laid down as muscle and how much as scar tissue—which is nothing more than disorganized, weak connective tissue—also is not clear. Muscle tissue, connective tissue, and scar tissue are three distinct categories to physiologists, but are not necessarily so clearly distinguished in real life. The hands-on therapists tend to suspect some kind of fibrosis as the culprit in muscle shortening: a literal turning of muscle fiber into connective fiber. It seems to happen mostly near the muscle ends, where muscle tissue gradually turns into tendon anyway. Hard use develops muscle tissue, but it may also slowly shift the area that divides muscle from tendon—not entirely distinct in any case—away from the joint and toward the muscle, reducing strength and increasing the risk of tendon injury. Athletes and trainers describe a muscle in that condition as "tight"—a sign that it is overused. Stretching has the unusual capacity to help turn scar tissue into more functional connective tissue. It helps resist any such shift.

This function implies another, much larger role of stretching in maintaining suppleness. If you've ever had a limb in a cast, you know how dramatically muscle tissue wastes away from lack of movement. Movement, or contraction, is what maintains muscle health. Tension—stretching—seems similarly to help maintain connective tissue health. Without regular contraction, muscle tissue atrophies; without regular tension, connective tissue loses its suppleness.

ANTISTRETCHING

Despite all this, and despite the almost universal (and successful) adoption of stretching programs by most serious athletic organizations, there is an antistretching lobby. For example, Dr. E. C. Frederick, director of research for Nike shoes, has made the argument that for distance running, no great range of motion is called for, and in fact a stiff muscle may be more efficient than a loose one, because of its greater passive tension. Frederick is a scientist, and a careful one, but his attention may be focused more intently on understanding performance than on finding ways to preserve it. In any event, he's not confident of the quality and soundness of the limited amount of research that has been done on stretching.

Neither is Dr. Richard H. Dominguez, a practicing orthopedist and author of *Total Body Training* (Warner Books, 1982). Dominguez says there's a "cult of flexibility" sweeping the country, made up of people who are trying to become contortionists. While he agrees that a certain amount of flexibility is a good thing, and stiffness isn't, he thinks that the would-be contortionists are doing themselves more harm than good: "In fact, every week we see more injuries from stretching than injuries that are a result of stiffness." He's quite vehement about the poor quality of research on stretching. (Too much of it, he points out, is done by graduate students to fulfill degree requirements, usually with very small samples of student-body subjects. It is not an inaccurate charge, and stretching is not the only aspect of exercise physiology to which it might be applied.) I haven't seen Dominguez's data demonstrating more injuries from stretching than from stiffness, or an explanation of how that distinction is made. One survey at a marathon in Hawaii a few years back did indicate that entrants who habitually stretched suffered more injuries than runners who didn't. The sampling procedure wasn't terribly scientific, but the antistretchers can always be depended upon to cite it.

In *Total Body Training*, Dominguez presents a "hit list" of stretching exercises that he considers dangerous, and makes a good case that they should be avoided. They include the yoga plow, the hurdler's stretch, duck walking and deep knee bends, toe touching, ballet stretches, and some others. (None is included in this book.) "If you can bend a joint beyond your ability to control it with muscle strength," he says, "you risk either tearing the muscles, tendons, or ligaments that support the joint, or damaging the joint surface itself through abnormal pressure upon it."

Can't argue with that. Some people stretch too hard. If you try too hard to do something, you're likely to hurt yourself. Don't hurt yourself: that's the first rule of stretching, I guess. I wouldn't have thought it needed to be stated, but perhaps it does. The professionals who would help us manage our bodies traditionally do not trust us not to hurt ourselves.

I am fascinated by this habit of what might be called scientificness. Stretching is an entirely natural and instinctive way of maintaining soft tissue health. It became controversial only when we started trying to codify it, to make it more scientific. We started constructing rules by which to stretch. (Don't bend your knees.) We began to get competitive at it. (I can stretch farther than you, and therefore am in some way better. One common test of physical fitness, sometimes administered even by health professionals, is the "sit and stretch" test, in which you sit flat-legged on the floor and measure how far you can reach toward or beyond your toes—i.e., if you have a competitive streak, find the point at which your hamstrings start to tear.) We began taking stretching's measrements. (See p. 107, Proprioceptive Neuromuscular Facilitation, a complex technique for increasing range of motion.) We began forbidding various forms of stretching, citing expertise, as in Dr. Dominguez's hit list, or the generally accepted ban against "ballistic" stretching.

Ballistic stretching is one of the terms—along with *stretch reflex* and *range of motion*—you can expect to hear anytime the subject of stretching comes up. It's a made-up term, intended to make stretching more scientific. Ballistics is the study of projectiles in flight. Exercise physiologists applied the term to movements that are started by a muscular contraction but completed by momentum, such as throwing and kicking. It's a vague enough concept: there's no indication of when muscular force must stop and momentum take over for the motion to become ballistic, or how much muscular control may be maintained in the completion phase. Someone must have noted that it sometimes hurts when you bob down quickly to touch your toes. The experts decided this was harmful, as it probably is, named such bouncing up and down *ballistic stretching,* and forbade it. All the authorities—both the prostretching and the antistretching lobbies—now agree that ballistic stretching is dangerous, a bad thing, inviting injury. Stop it, you're going to hurt yourself.

Serious athletes, however, who have to learn their own most effective ways of managing their bodies, still use ballistic stretching (formerly known as calisthenics) when warming up. They do a little of that along with a little of everything else—some loose, jiggly jogging, a burst of power now and then, an increasingly quick rehearsal of the moves to come, but always, in between each move, the slow, easy stretching out of things. Uncodified. When the athlete begins bobbing in the middle of a stretch, the authorities wince, and predict disaster. They don't trust experienced athletes, either. The athletes continue with what works. Sure enough, sometimes they do injure themselves. (While I was working on this book, the wire services reported that Montreal Expos conditioning coach Bill Sellers, in spring training, tore a hamstring—while stretching.)

Looking to science for backing, the codifiers have invoked the "stretch reflex" as the villain in ballistic stretching. The stretch reflex is the mechanism that put the term *knee-jerk* into the language. When the doctor taps your kneecap (actually, your patellar tendon), the force yanks on the tendon, which stretches a receptor and fires its nerve, telling the spinal cord to contract the thigh muscle attached to the tendon. When that muscle contracts, it jerks your foot forward, assuring the doctor that your wiring is intact.

The codifiers reasoned that if you yank on a muscle by stretching it "ballistically"—bobbing against the end of its tendon—the stretch reflex will contract the muscle so you're stretching against a contraction, and you may tear something. A slow stretch, with the tension held steady for twenty seconds, is alleged to bypass the stretch reflex.

I'm not sure about this. It's not bad advice. Bouncing up and down on the limits of your hamstrings isn't very smart. Neither is any other forceful move against tight tissue, at whatever speed of application. The slower the move, the more control you have. Whether you have to hold each move for twenty seconds and then take up the slack, whether you are in fact bypassing the stretch reflex, whether it's even a bad idea to stretch against a contraction—I'm not sure of any of that. Forcing a muscle to lengthen *quickly* against a contraction puts the heaviest load on it that it ever undergoes. (Imagine you're moving a heavy sofa, and someone suddenly jumps on your end.) But that doesn't mean you can't safely pull a muscle out to greater length while it is resisting the pull. That's called an *eccentric contraction*—"yielding work" —which you use every time you lower a load or walk downhill. If it were dangerous, approximately half of all human movement would put us at risk.

Similarly, the stretching experts propose an almost fetishist pursuit of range of motion—which turns out to be as fuzzy a notion as ballistic stretching. Increased range of motion is the very thing for which we are supposed to be stretching. If only we knew what it means. Sometimes range of motion means the maximum angle in any direction that the mechanical structure of the joint will permit the limb or body segment to assume, or the anatomical limits to passive joint motion: how far someone can move your relaxed limb. At other times, the term is used to mean the difference between the maximum stretched length of the muscle and the minimum contracted length of the muscle, which determines the maximum distance the skeletal segment can be moved actively by its own muscle: how far you can move your own limb.

If you're stretching to increase the first kind of range of motion—against anatomical limits—then you may well be risking structural damage. That kind of stretching is what I presume Dr. Dominguez is concerned about, and it does sound like a dubious practice. But if you're stretching to keep muscle and connective tissue long and loose, to maintain their maximum active, useful length, then you're maintaining soft tissue health. If that's a bad idea, then so is all exercise, all activity, all human motion.

INTERNAL STRETCHING

There is one aspect of stretching about which all are in agreement. You do want to relax as much as possible the muscle tissue you're stretching. No controversy here: stretching should be an aid to relaxation in every way, a de-tensifier, a gentle wringing out of all our strictures and contractions, muscular or otherwise.

A powerful tool for relaxation is the deep breath. Most presentations of stretching emphasize breathing as an adjunct to every stretch, often venturing into anatomical looniness to do so. (Breathe *into* the stretch. Direct your breathing into your calf muscle as you stretch it. Breathe through the top of your head.) If the image works for you—if you can follow the advice without giggling—then it's probably a useful tool.

It's probably a good idea even if you do break into giggles: Norman Cousins points out that laughter is a way of taking your internal organs out for a jog. Laughing stretches the diaphragm, just as a good deep breath does. Smiling and laughing give the facial musculature a good stretch. (Yoga has you making horrific faces to accomplish the same thing.) There are plenty of other nonmusculoskeletal aspects of our physiology for which a good stretch is an effective toner, if you can just figure a way of getting at them to stretch them out.

Deep breathing is one of the best. A good deep breath may be the most powerful natural tranquilizer available to us, the system's own miracle drug, the universal palliative. All creatures call upon its restorative powers. Horses and dogs definitely do; I think I've even heard a chicken sigh. In times of stress we air-breathers want at least one chest-expanding, inhale-plus-exhale before plunging into the action, whether the action is swinging at a fastball, skiing an icy mogul field, or uttering the opening line of a public speech. Experienced performers take such breaths consciously, deliberately calling on deep breathing's powers of relaxation. When the circumstances are severe enough—when we are sufficiently uncertain about impending events—the same settling inhale/exhale will be wrenched from us, whatever our level of experience. The body, in its wisdom, demands it.

In yoga almost as much attention is devoted to breath control as to stretching. Special ways of breathing are aimed at centering and calming the body, to free the mind for higher pursuits. Stress-reduction clinics often start with breath control before they go on to all that Type A and Type B stuff. Counting to ten when you lose your temper—folk wisdom's sound advice—is in part a delay to give you a couple of breaths to get hold of yourself.

Personally, I've found deep breathing to be a nearly perfect sleeping pill. As I settle down to sleep I deliberately take and hold a deep "belly" breath, pushing my stomach out and downward as I expand my chest, consciously stretching the diaphragm—which is all muscle and connective tissue—for a few seconds. I then exhale fully, close my windpipe, and suck my gut back toward my spine, stretching the diaphragm in the other direction. I take another deep breath and relax everything, and about thirty seconds later I fall asleep. My wife points out that I do the same without these exercises, but that's an unscientific, subjective observation.

I am convinced that there is physiology for this phenomenon—stretch receptors in the diaphragm, most likely, activation of which releases tranquilizing biochemicals. Science has not, that I know of, identified these stretch receptors and brain chemicals, but that's okay. Even if it's just a placebo response, the process puts me to sleep anyway.

STRETCHERS VS. NONSTRETCHERS

The controversies over stretching aren't the product of science but of its lack. There isn't sufficient evidence for either side to make its case. Each of the two sides, pro- and antistretching, finds the opposite position incomprehensible. As is usually the case when disagreement is so direct, a certain emotional tone sneaks into the discussion, indicating that something other than fact is at work in these matters.

The disagreement probably has less to do with science and evidence than either side will admit. I think there are simply people who like the feel of stretching, and people who don't, and that all the rationales for either side are to support subjective reaction to particular physical sensations. People who don't like to stretch don't like the way it feels. They find it frightening, somehow, or at least nervous-making, to feel that electric crackle of a fully extended muscle-tendon unit. (There are also people who are made nervous by sex.) Perhaps this book, being about pleasure, isn't for those people.

All the science in the world isn't going to turn them into enthusiastic stretchers; maybe nothing can accomplish that. But I hope they understand that there's a way to go at stretching that bypasses all of that curious argumentation and pseudoscience, and that it doesn't require stop watches or any other form of measurement. Stretching is a progression, which you can stop at any point. There's no reason, scientific or otherwise, not to keep it pleasurable.

THREE

HOW TO
WORK OUT

There is a popular literature of stretching, a veritable stream of how-to books and magazine articles that purport to guide you through the basic principles. They're not exactly wrong, but I find them shortsighted, and frustrating to use. They tend to be rigidly doctrinaire, which strikes me as a peculiar way to approach the subject of flexibility.

For example, most of the stretching literature insists that you warm up before you stretch. It's a chicken-or-egg question. Certainly, muscle and connective tissue accept tension better when they're at a proper operating temperature and well supplied with blood. On the other hand, they also accept warming up better if they're already stretched out to length, loose and supple. You have to start somewhere. Stretching is one way of warming up. Warming up before you stretch is fine if it works for you. As doctrine it is of a piece with the advice never to stretch ballistically: if you try to yank cold muscles and tendons out to length, you can hurt yourself. Don't hurt yourself. That's sound stretching advice.

(Personally, I stretch a little, warm up a little, stretch some more. Before and after the hard part of any workout, I check my frame for specific stiffnesses and stretch those areas. But the best, concentrated stretching comes at the end of the day, when I am less distracted.)

Most stretching texts also tell you to stretch as far as is

comfortable, hold the stretch for twenty or thirty seconds, then take up the slack for another thirty seconds or so. This time sequence is proposed to give the stretch reflex time to "relax." But the stretch reflex isn't a muscle, it's a neural signal, in immediate response to sudden tension. The stretch reflex doesn't have anything to do with the slow, progressive, therapeutic stretching out of soft tissue, it just sounds as if it should be, so the stretching manuals talk about it a lot.

Furthermore, forty to sixty seconds per stretch means that a thorough stretching program—particularly if done before and after hard work—would take more time than most workouts last. This promotes the tendency to settle for a perfunctory stretch of the big muscles and let everything else go. That's what happens when you get doctrinaire about a process that should be slow and easy, that's done by feel, not by numbers.

In fact most current stretching advice is generated by the same quick-fix mentality that prescribes exercise as dosage: thirty minutes of elevated heart rate, taken once per day, a magic bullet against the ills of modern-day life. Most runners are runners not because they love to run but because that's the simplest and quickest way to get the exercise dosage out of the way. (Serious runners are often people who started that way, then discovered a taste for the sport—or a talent—and so made room in their schedules for their special passion.)

Consider a typical run. Most of us don exercise gear, step out the door, and are gone—promising ourselves, usually, to use the first mile as a warm-up. The more guilt-ridden may pause to swing one foot up against a wall and stretch out the hamstring (the riskiest and least effective way to do so). Maybe we'll stretch the front of the thigh, lean against a wall and pull on the calf a bit; if we're feeling particularly stiff we may spread-eagle and bend alternate knees, stretching out the groin. That's about it. If we're extraordinarily meticulous, we'll stop after a mile or so and repeat at least some of this brief routine after we're warmed up. If we're obsessive-compulsive, we'll go through it again when we finish the run, before showering. Done: with a little practice, we can be dressed and back to our busy lives before our heart rates drop back to normal.

It's not a bad routine; we can get away with it for a long time if we keep the mileage low, if we're young and resilient, if we don't slip or stumble into trauma, if we don't do any other strenuous thing beyond our daily run. To the degree that we bother with that sort of brief regular stretching program, we probably reduce the chance of injury, or at least postpone it. But it's not going to keep us supple. To achieve that, we have to think a little differently about working out, and about stretching. We have to change the way we use time.

STRETCHING IT OUT

You already know how to stretch. You're an expert at it. Even if you live a completely sedentary life, you stretch every day, habitually and safely. You stretch whenever your body demands it, which is usually when you haven't been moving around enough for the body's tastes. You also stretch after you've been moving too much.

You stretch automatically, reflexively. When you get up from your desk, your theater seat, even from your comfortable bed, you stretch out exactly those parts that want stretching the most; they tell you to stretch them, and you comply. In order to ease your stiffness, you *move* things, slowly, more or less gently, pulling taut your lower back, trunk, shoulders, neck. Doing so usually makes you yawn—reflexively—which stretches your jaw and face. It makes you groan with pleasure. You stretch what feels good, for as long as it feels good to do so. This rule was given to me by my son, and in fact is the only rigid rule you'll find in this book. It bears repeating: Stretch only what feels good, for as long as it feels good to do so. Afterward, what you will feel is relief.

All the principles of a successful stretching program are contained above. To increase the pleasure, and the relief, you'll only be ringing variations on those principles, expanding their application. That takes a little experimentation, a little feeling around in the musculoskeletal system to find what works best for you. You may also have to learn to think a little differently about what you're doing. You have to learn to experience your body as a single piece.

Try an experiment. Let your hand rest on some solid surface. Begin pushing down as if you're trying to push that surface through the floor. Slowly increase the pressure. Feel the muscular contraction work its way up, starting at your wrist, progressing up the forearm and the back of the upper arm. (Feel how slack the biceps has gone, almost toneless, as you tighten the triceps: that's *reciprocal inhibition*, another reflex.)

You feel this progressive contraction first as a stiffening of the wrist joint and then the elbow, the smaller muscles locking the joint into immobility before the larger muscles are brought into play and real force is exerted. If you continue to bear down, you'll draw tight a complex arrangement of muscles and tendons around the shoulder joint, locking it tight too. Continue, and as you run out of available increase from the obvious large muscles of arm and shoulder, you will bring in musculature of the chest and back, searching for ways to apply your body weight to that downward-pressing palm.

This small experiment demonstrates several things about the stretching process. It illuminates, for example, the intricacy of the structures involved in generating real force. The large muscles—biceps, triceps, thighs, hamstrings, calves—dominate our athletic thinking, but they can't be put to work until complex systems of smaller muscle-tendon units have braced and aligned the frame and properly set the joints. We direct our training and our maintenance to the major muscles, assuming that the peripheral structures will take care of themselves. But soreness and injuries occur in muscles we don't perceive as major, and do so perhaps more frequently than they do in the larger, stronger structures. Those "minor" injuries put us out of action as effectively as do mishaps to the big stuff.

It's also worth noting how that ripple of contraction spreads from your palm throughout your body. As you keep increasing the downward force, the sensation is as if you're drawing tight a net—one that extends from your palm right on throughout the rest of your body, head to toes. You won't feel it pull tight everywhere, even if you really get serious about increasing the force, but apply enough pressure and you will feel it pull in all directions. You can trace it around joints, across your back, even down the backs of your legs. This is the network that ties you into a single anatomical piece. This network of muscle and connective tissue is what you want to learn to stretch back out to length.

Also worth considering is how you search around in your anatomy for ways to increase the force. It's almost as if you are trying and discarding various elements—muscles, angles, ways of getting an anatomical purchase on the problem—to find what works best. You'll find yourself using this same kind of conscious search through the anatomy as you invent new ways to stretch. With it you'll find no end of new places, new parts of yourself, that are accessible to stretching, that in fact cry out for it. If there is a single tool that makes for a successful stretching program, it is this level of attention. Zen Buddhists must be talking about something very like this when they speak of "one-pointedness."*

This is not the same kind of attention you use for ordinary athletic effort. If the athletic task is to put more downward force on your hand, you won't be thinking about anything but that force; your central nervous system or your coordination or your innate body sense conducts the search, throwing everything it can find into the task. There is seldom time, in the athletic moment, to consider anatomical alternatives that might better achieve your aim. But in the thoughtful and considered effort of the preceding experiment—and in the similar intentional awareness of a good

---

*When hauling water, the Zen master says, just haul water; when chopping wood, just chop wood. That is, don't haul around your problems with the IRS, don't chop up your boss along with the wood. When stretching, just stretch—but pay attention.

stretch—you have the opportunity to find and familiarize yourself with the complex ways your musculoskeletal system ties together. A good stretch is always an anatomy lesson. The more of your anatomy you fully understand—not from anatomy charts but experientially, from day-to-day work with its fine detail—the more of it you have available to conscious control. The clearer your sense of your anatomy, the better (and safer) your athletic efforts will be.

The clearer your sense of your anatomy, the more pleasure and relaxation you will get out of stretching. If you only stretch reflexively, unconsciously, as when you rise from your desk, you're working with mere tissue. If you stretch consciously, reading the sensations and using them to guide your movements, you are held, for brief moments, anyway, in the present tense. Spending time in the present tense, instead of restlessly reevaluating the past or worrying about the future, is the deepest rest there is. That, too, is a kind of one-pointedness, a way of capturing a bit of time for yourself and getting maximum use from it.

THE PLEASURE PART

You want to hold each stretch just as long as it holds your attention. When your mind begins to wander, stretch something else. You definitely don't want to rush. You want a relaxed and leisurely approach, a sense of taking the pressure off. Stretching should, in effect, unplug your phone. It should be a signal to your brain: Let go, damn it. Step out of your Type A life (or the Type A aspects of your life) for a little while. Drop your tensed shoulders, ease off that cramp at the back of your neck. Kick off your metaphorical shoes, even if you're already barefoot.

Relaxation is what you're after; you pursue it by applying, then letting go of, tension. You are as interested in relaxing the contractility of the muscle as you are in pulling taut the elasticity of its tendons. Focusing your mind on what's happening, making sure you've let everything go in the muscle, does take a little while, in every stretch. This is time you fill with gradually increasing tension.* It's not a bad idea to hold a given tension, then take up the slack. Your guide shouldn't be a fixed number of seconds, however, but the sensation you're getting from the elements you're stretching. If you're stretching your hamstring, you should feel the fibers pull tight behind the knee at first, then, as you increase pressure, from heel to butt along the back of your leg. Pay attention to that progression. I find that if I really concentrate, I can almost always find a little something else in there to relax, another fraction of an inch of movement to pick up. Another notch forward. That conscious relaxation, that focus on the area you're stretching, seems to do as much good as the actual lengthening of the tissue.

Reverse the experiment described on p. 28. Relax the downward force on your palm, and push your shoulder and elbow forward so you bend your wrist back, until you feel the connective tissue in the palm and the underside of your wrist begin to pull tight. Push your elbow farther forward and the tension works its way from wrist to palm to fingers to fingertips. This is an area of tissue that usually does not get stretched, which makes it easier to pay fresh attention to. You want to figure out how to make stretching it pleasurable.

You do that by experimenting with the level of tension. At the first level of tightness it has a familiar muscular feel to it; as you increase the tension it begins to feel as if nerves are involved: more tingly, electrical. There is a continuum of sensation from the initial tightness, relief of which is purely pleasurable, right on into pain. It is a continuum with which you want to become intimately familiar. In the earliest stages, you are taking out the slack, pulling things back out to their normal resting length. As you increase the tension, you begin to *work* the tissues, to pull fibers into alignment. That's when you begin to stimulate the

---

*How do you relax and apply tension at the same time? You relax the area you're stretching, and stretch it by pulling on it with other muscles. When you stretch your arms wide upon arising, for example, you contract the muscles across your back and shoulders in order to stretch your chest and the front of your shoulders.

biochemical processes that lead to actual growth, strengthening, improvement. Think of it that way: you're not yanking on the tissue or even trying literally to lengthen it, you're organizing it.

Apply too much tension and you begin to disrupt the tissue's own internal connections, to generate the microtrauma of hard use. Your guide to proper tension is pleasure: you want to learn to take the tension up the scale of intensity, without tipping over into the pain that signals that healing will have to take place. You never want to stretch anything harder than you stretch your arms and back when you climb out of bed in the morning. (If you feel you have to stretch it hard, you haven't got the correct angle of pull. Feel around, try some other angles, find a way to put gentle tension on it in a controllable manner.)

Stretching your hand and forearm is a useful test for familiarizing yourself with these sensations. Unless you are a pianist or violinist, or otherwise use those parts of your anatomy long and hard, you won't often be inclined to stretch them out. You may find you can do so more effectively by pressing your hands palm to palm, or locking your fingers, palms outward, and straightening your elbows, in the time-honored pianist's limbering-up routine. But leaning on one hand on a table and pressing the elbow forward to stretch fingers, palm, wrist, and forearm is a nicely controllable way to experiment with stretching tensions and their sensations.

Once you have a sense of the level of tension that begins to work the tissue, try twisting from side to side at the wrist, or rolling your elbow from one side to the other. Rotate the bones gently against each other. This stretch extends the wrist; try flexing it, stretching it in the opposite direction, reaching back toward the elbow with the fingertips. You're working an extremely complex structure: nineteen major bones in the fingers and hand alone, eight more in the wrist, two in the forearm, all tied together with distinctive ligaments, worked by separate sets of muscles for flexing and for extending, each muscle attached to the bone by tendons on each end.

All of these structures need movement to maintain their health.

Work them too little and the connective tissue begins to deteriorate, the joints to lose their mobility (the onset of degenerative joint disease); work them too much and they accumulate the biochemical and structural results of fatigue. They need the healthy tension of stretching to set things right again. Musicians, artists, even assembly-line workers who use their hands very hard, suffer crippling overuse injuries when they lose the suppleness of their hands. Careful warm-up by flexing—mostly in the form of gentle stretching—is how suppleness is maintained. A little exploration will quickly turn up half a dozen other ways to flex these intricate structures. One of the best is simply to spread your fingers wide, stiffening and extending hands and fingers. Hold the extension stiffly for a few seconds, and you'll begin to feel muscular fatigue too—and you can begin to compare that sensation with the sensation of a good stretch. You'll want to be able to distinguish between the two. People who don't stretch seem to have trouble doing so.

THE SENSATION

At the end of a hard day you may often get the frustrating feeling that somewhere in the middle of your back there's a place where one good crack, one adjustment (in the chiropractic sense), would cure everything: all that pent-up, loaded tension in there would finally find a way to release itself. Stretching it out helps—and in fact is the only way you can usually find to ease that knot of tension—but it's hard to avoid the sense that it would all go away with just the right move.

Similarly, from time to time you'll get the sense that if you only stretched a little harder, something important would finally click into place, some important function would be restored. You'd be healed, somehow, completely freed up.

That's how to make stretching dangerous. The feeling is delusional, of course. Nothing *is* going to click into place (but you can tear tissue). Getting and staying supple is a slow, steady process, just like any other kind of physical training, just like the increase in muscle size that comes from strength training. You can't do it all in one workout. Elite athletes and their coaches all agree that the single most important mental attribute you bring to any kind of training is patience.

What you can do, during and after every workout, is return the tissue to its best possible state, put it back the way it ought to be: stretched loose, cleaned out, freshened up for more use. Every workout should start with the tissues in this neutral but ready state. Then, when you get them warm and pumping with fluids, lubricated and well nourished, you can start working on them, pushing them farther in whatever direction your training program wants to take them. After you've finished, you want to put them back in the neutral state. To do this carefully and systematically is to ratchet yourself one click farther, in effect, in the direction of suppleness.

It is from these principles that you want to design your personal soft-tissue maintenance program. A workout can and perhaps needs to be fast and hard, a stint of aggressive effort designed to wring out your physical systems thoroughly, to take you well into the realm of temporary fatigue. Stress the systems and then allow them to recover; that's how you gain. But wrapped around every workout should be some slow time, some quiet, introspective attention paid to the musculoskeletal state of things. You want to switch gears for that, take the pressure off.

You'll find what works for you, what you have time for. You should at least try to check for unusual stiffness before you start any workout, and this requires a certain amount of full extension of the joints. (If movement in one direction feels stiff, pay particular attention to stretching the muscle group that moves the limb in the opposite direction.) You'll want to monitor your warm-up carefully, and your cool-down should also be conscientious: an abrupt halt to hard exercise is nearly as hard on your system as too abrupt a beginning.

You probably won't feel you have time for a systematic stretching-out at the end of every workout. If something feels sore or tight, you'll pay it some attention, but you won't put every-thing exactly right every time. That's all right. (Guilt, too, is bad for suppleness.) But whatever your exercise routine, keep in mind that recovery time is as important a part of training as is progres-sive loading. You'll want to follow every hard training day with an easy day, and the easy days should be devoted to maintenance, rather than hard use, of soft tissue. The goal is to spend the easy workouts in a quiet cocoon of attention to detail, to the state of things as you bring them up to operating temperature and then burn off a little energy. That's when you can find time to work things back out to length, pull out the sorenesses. Work them, but don't stress them: easy days are for learning—and practicing—the difference.

As you accustom yourself to regular stretching, you'll proba-bly find that in between workouts, as you go about the routine of your daily life, you'll start doing a lot of musculoskeletal monitor-ing. You'll come to recognize how a momentary fatigue or stiffness anywhere can be stretched out, casually and unobtrusively. You'll learn lots of little tricks for doing so—sitting in chairs, standing in doorways, you'll find a way to shift your weight, get a small purchase on something solid, and pull taut this long muscle or that one, relieving it. Refreshing it. It is a day-long antidote against the unnaturalness of sitting still. Nobody need ever notice.

(As I work, I stretch out my arms, neck, and shoulders every half-hour or so. I was probably doing it anyway, unconsciously, long before I started stretching, but now I do it consciously and, I admit, addictively. It helps an enormous amount: I finish the day without the knots and glitches that used to have me groaning with fatigue by quitting time.)

Eventually, every day, whether you've worked out or not, you'll find yourself going through some version of the moves described in chapter 4. I do mine at night. I change into soft clothing—sweats, of course—and drop a small mat on the floor during the late news. I then spend an utterly relaxing half-hour there, simply writhing; there's no better word for it. Working my way slowly and methodically through the accessible muscle groups, stretching everything out to length, getting long and loose again before sleep. Putting things back in order for the next day. I may miss a day or two now and then for travel, a deadline, social obligations. But after about forty-eight hours without stretching, my body refuses to be ignored any longer. It seizes me by the back of the neck and throws me down on the floor, crying, "Stretch me!" I follow its instructions. Delicious.

The popular stretching manuals give you lists of *don'ts*. I'm not sure that is necessary. There are a couple of stretching positions that are ill advised because they're hard to control, and if you lose control you can hurt yourself. Hurting yourself certainly should be forbidden, I agree with that. But the only other practice that I would forbid is competitive stretching. That's why I don't like the idea of group stretching exercises. I think stretching is best done in private.

A distressing number of runners stretch only if other runners (or photographers) are around; some of them admit it. If you stretch in public, you will be tempted to demonstrate how flexible you are, particularly if you're warming up around other exercisers. If you're stretching in a group, the same temptation will apply. If you have a group leader, a stretching guru, you'll want to show that person how well you are following instructions. I don't care how oblivious to the rest of the world you think you are, if other people are around, you'll stretch harder, reach farther, than if you're by yourself. You can't help it, it's just the way the human animal works.

It might help to consider that what you're actually demonstrating is not some mysterious athletic capacity or moral virtue but a particular arrangement of bones, joint angles, and tissue lengths: a set of dimensions. That you can reach your toes with your knees locked doesn't mean you are slimmer or faster or better trained than someone who can't; it means that your hamstrings are longer. Being proud of long hamstrings makes about as much sense as being proud of a long nose. The fellow who can't reach past his knees may have healthier, more supple hamstrings than the guy who can touch his elbows to his toes, if that's the way each happens to be built.

The point of stretching isn't to see (or show) how far you can reach, or even to reach as far as you can, but to pull the tissues out to length and put a little healthy tension on them. A *little*. To accomplish that, you have to pay attention. You can pay attention better in private.

Back to the sensation, for a moment—the tingling, more or less electrified feeling that you're working with when you stretch. What you're feeling is the firing of thousands of nerve endings. These are nerve endings in the richly innervated connective tissue that are specifically structured to be activated *by* stretching.

I like to think of them as signaling the connective tissue to stay alive. Connective tissue, like muscle, is kept healthy by the signals for work. It is the firing of nerve endings that keeps the transactions going on—the laying down of new fiber and the arrangement of it into healthy tissue, the exchanges of biochemistry, the lubrication and nutrition and waste removal. What you feel when you stretch is the care and feeding of your connective tissue.

Ordinary exercise also fires these nerve endings, of course, but tends to do so too specifically. Too much connective tissue, in the immense complexity of our muscular structure, is ignored or bypassed; the rest—the readily accessible and narrowly activated—is all too often overused. Stretching is the tool for bringing the level of use back into the happy middle ground.

THE MOVES

Friends ask me to show them stretches, but I can't really do that: a position isn't a stretch, it's more complicated than that. That's what this book is for. But once you grasp the principles, stretching is not so much complicated as it is wonderfully rich with possibilities. The moves that follow should give you a glimpse of those possibilities.

They are starting points for a thorough stretching program, but starting points only: they are not etched in stone. As you explore your own one-piece anatomy, you'll invent better—more pleasurable—moves of your own. These are intended only to give you a point of entry, so to speak, for stretching the major areas of soft tissue.

You can do them on the floor, on the ground, even on a firm bed. Most are done lying down, and a little padding makes things more comfortable. I keep a small exercise mat handy. Stretching while you're standing makes it harder to relax, harder to maintain your balance and control the amount of tension. Runners and other outdoor, damp-ground exercisers may nevertheless prefer to stand. That's okay—you can adapt some of these moves to standing positions, and you'll surely invent substitutes for the ones you can't. [Note: All of the exercises in this book should be done gently, without the use of excessive force. Readers who have not previously engaged in a regular exercise program, or who have musculoskeletal problems or have suffered musculoskeletal injuries, should see a doctor first, and should proceed with caution.]

However you do the moves, you'll want to wear some kind of loose clothing (or none at all). A towel or a three-foot length of surgical tubing makes a useful stretching tool, extending your reach, expanding the possibilities. The only other equipment you'll need is a relaxed frame of mind—and if you don't have that when you start a stretching session, you should by the time you finish.

More rigid approaches to stretching make a big thing about the order of progression. I'm not sure how important that is, but it seems logical to begin with the center of the body—the trunk—and proceed limbward. With the exception of the first two, that's the way these moves are presented. (I like to imagine that I'm chasing my stiffness from the center outward, as if chasing air bubbles out from under contact paper. Imagery seems to help concentration. When the therapist or masseur tells you to "breathe into" the area being worked on, the image is supposed to help you relax the affected muscles.)

What follows are moves, not positions: there's nothing static about them. In each case you'll want to assume your own comfortable version of the illustration, and then begin, gently, to work with it—to exaggerate it, to move it from side to side, to discover how you can change the angle at which the tension is applied. You want to pull against whatever feels tight, enjoying how the sensation builds with the tension. You'll find yourself stopping from time to time, holding a given position for long enough for the sensation to stabilize, then resuming tension. Sometimes it helps to back off tension completely, move the joint a bit to explore its level of tightness, and then stretch it again.

When you've stretched a given area sufficiently, the pleasure starts to subside. When that happens, changing position slightly—bringing new tissue under tension—can bring back the sensation of a fruitful stretch. That's the key to pleasurable stretching: recognition of what a good stretch feels like, when it is over, and where you have to go, anatomically, to bring back the pleasure.

When a stretch feels finished, for example, you can usually enhance or renew it by merely inclining your head a bit in one direction or another, stretching the neck, pulling into tension just a little more of the body's one-piece connective net.

At its most effective and most pleasurable, stretching is a meditative interlude, a productive place to put the mind for a while. The teaching of meditation isn't the purpose here, but the result sought by most meditative disciplines—the unkinking of the psyche, so to speak—is not that different from that of a good stretch. Stretching works on the physical instead of the mental plane, but therefore works a lot more concretely than mental practices ever can. The sensation of stretching—the signal from the tissues—can be a powerful aid to mental focus, drawing your attention back, with every increase in tension, to the site and the process. And as meditation also demonstrates, paying that kind of attention is the route to the deepest (most pleasurable) level of result.

There's plenty for the mind to focus on, if only in what is transpiring physically in the muscle and connective tissue as you stretch it. The more or less exhaustive anatomical detail in the following chapters is intended in part to make sure you have plenty to mull over while you go through these moves. The transactions described—the straightening of fibers, the flushing of wastes, the quieting of neuromuscular noise—are in fact happening as you stretch. I find it nicely reaffirming, somehow, to contemplate these mechanisms while they're at work. I enjoy trying to connect signal to image: Oh, I find myself saying, so *that's* what that feels like.

You can also profitably trace attachment points—which will surprise you now and then—and contemplate lines of force. (That's how stretching teaches anatomy.) Big muscles are easiest to stretch. As it happens, the masses of tissue that you can stretch most directly are generally the masses of tissue through which you are able to generate the most force. The "dead lift," for example (forget about style, let's just see how much pure weight you can get off the ground), is the most purely forceful human activity I can think of. It makes primary use of the capacity to extend the legs, hips, and back, because that's where our maximum power lies. That's also where we're most accessible to stretching. What can pull powerfully and directly can be pulled *on* powerfully and directly.

Weightlifting doesn't seem like "pulling," but as they say in physics, you can't push on a rope. Muscles don't push. Even when you're shoving a car out of a ditch, your muscles are pulling. Think of the common push-up: your muscles aren't pushing against the floor but trying to straighten the arm by pulling on the bones. The triceps, at the back of the upper arm, pulls around the corner—across the joint—of the elbow; the forearm muscles extend the wrist. The same is true of any move you make. To understand stretching, it is important to understand this. The only thing any muscle can do is contract; all stretching is aimed at pulling it back out to its proper length.

Big, simple motions use big, simple muscles. It is when you get to more complex and awkward activities, and the muscles and tendons that are used for them, that the stretching gets complex and awkward. We generally allow our shoulders and arms to specialize in complex and awkward tasks (unless we're soccer players). Figuring out how to stretch out all the muscles and tendons used in throwing, say, or swimming, is an anatomical jigsaw puzzle.

The way you solve such puzzles is not by flipping through these pages in search of just the right position, but by finding out where you can go from the positions illustrated: not by stretching in static positions but by moving from position to position, stretching everything in between as you go. You do this by what I can only call rolling around the joint: putting a stretching tension on a limb or body segment and then revolving the angle of force through as many degrees of arc as body structure allows. Once you get a feel for this technique, you can virtually move the stretch from muscle-tendon unit to muscle-tendon unit through 360 degrees around the joint.

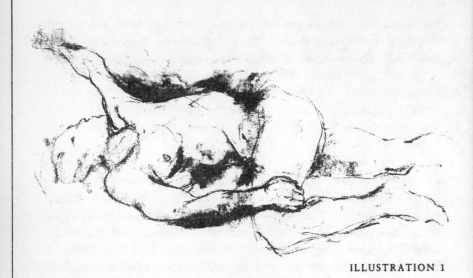

ILLUSTRATION 1

One of my favorite stretches is simply to lie on one side and slowly circle my other, relaxed arm in as wide an arc as the joint allows. To do so not only stretches out the complex structure of muscles and tendons on the front side of the shoulder joint but begins to work on the upper back, the rib cage, and the breast muscles.* The weight of hand and arm usually provides enough tension; if it doesn't, and I find a particularly productive segment of the arc, I'll grab the underside of a door or a piece of furniture and roll my body away slightly to increase the tension. (If needed, I'll use a towel or elastic tubing to extend my reach.)

The first sensation is of stretching out the moderate-sized muscles and tendons around the shoulder joint. As you continue, increasing the tension and reaching for a little deeper stretch,

---

*For the back of the shoulder joint—*posterior deltoid, trapezius, rhomboids,* and their multitude of tendons—you'll have better results starting from illustration 18. Where possible, I've tried to use common and familiar anatomical terms here—"calf," rather than *gastrocnemius.* Readers who already know their gastrocnemius won't be misled, and those who haven't memorized all that Latin won't be driven to *Gray's Anatomy.* Where the proper anatomical name is needed, I've tried to describe the area in familiar terms.

you'll begin to feel the pull on the great sheets of connective tissue that bind shoulder muscles into the breast and upper back, which reach across the trunk to the opposite hip. (It is stretching these large sheets of tissue, called *fascia*, that is most satisfying to me, that feels as if it's doing the most good. Stretching the tissues of the breast, incidentally—the pectoral region—is much neglected. If your shoulders slump, maybe it isn't a moral failure—sorry, Mom—or that your back is tired or weak, but that your breast is too tight. Such tightness, over the years, can put a permanent curve in your back. Anatomy *is* mutable.) As you work beyond the large sheets of fascia, increasing the tension and the angle, you begin to work the joint capsule itself, feeling out the limits of the joint's excursion. This progression—muscle to tendon to joint—is the goal in every stretch.

Stretching the shoulder through its range of motion also demonstrates the necessity for gentleness. You won't be able to move your arm smoothly through the entire arc. There are bony obstructions in the joint; to continue, you have to back off the tension and rotate your relaxed arm within its socket to clear them. You'll feel tendons slide over bone ends, and you may hear some alarming snaps or pops, particularly if you're moving too briskly. If you're putting too much pressure on the joint, those transactions won't be pleasant—they'll feel fishy and a little disconcerting, if not actually painful.

Working your way past these obstructions is an object lesson in the etiology and dynamics of overuse injuries: what you're feeling is tendinitis trying to be born. You're not going to give yourself tendinitis by easing your way around the joint's architecture in gentle stretching, but that kind of motion repeated in the heat of athletic effort is another matter. When a tendon slips over the knob of a bone under high tension, its blood supply is momentarily squeezed out of that area, interrupting its food supply. Its fibers, designed only for lengthwise tension, are subjected to fraying pressure. Healthy tendons can withstand a great deal of this treatment, but they have their limits. That's why, for example, the pitching coach counts his ballplayer's pitches. The notorious rotator cuff is a complex group of muscle-tendon units particularly vulnerable to this kind of fatigue.

Once the immediate shoulder-joint tissues feel loose, there are a couple of other places to go with this stretch. Make sure your top knee is raised so that the thigh is at a right angle to your body, your weight split between your side and your raised knee. As you reach back with arm and hand, try to keep your knee on the floor. Feel the stretching tension work from the shoulder joint to the breast to the trunk, twisting the spine, stretching out the lower back. By increasing or decreasing the angle of the knee as you move the arm, you can work the stretch up and down the spine, as well as throughout the rib cage, breast, and shoulder.

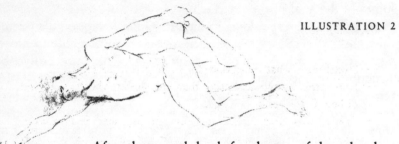

ILLUSTRATION 2

After that, reach back for the toe of the other leg. From this position, you can find half a dozen more productive stretches. Pull on the toe, relax the leg, and you'll stretch foot, shin (an antidote for shin splints), the front of the thigh, the hip, and the groin. By pulling the toe from one side to the other, you rotate the thigh bone in its hip socket, reaffirming its range of motion. Without changing position, switch your attention to your arm, and you'll find that by pulling with your lower leg instead of with your arm, you can stretch shoulder and breast in a little different way. By switching the stretching tension (and the relaxation) from arm to leg and back again, you can keep varying the stretch, searching out new angles, additional nooks and crannies of your anatomy that will welcome the attention. After you've run out of places to stretch, repeat with the other shoulder.

This is what I mean by rolling around the joint. It is a process of exploring, with tension, the angles through which the joint will work, the muscles and tendons that are involved in those angles, and the sheets of connective tissue that tie that joint into all the rest of the anatomy. And of stretching all of the above back out to their loose and comfortable resting lengths.

THE PROGRAM

Here's a sensible and easy-to-remember order of procedure, and some suggested moves. There are only six stretches—or six starting points, rather—for the basic program. (You'll invent others as you go.)

REMEMBER:

- Stretch only what feels good, for as long as it feels good.
- Don't stretch anything harder than you stretch when you get out of bed. Pain does not feel good.
- Try to work from muscle to tendon to ligament: from muscle-tendon unit to joint capsule.* And go easy on the ligament/joint capsule. Then seek out the sheets of fascia of the supporting musculature.
- If you are in doubt about whether something is right for you, talk to your doctor.

After you've been through the following moves a few times, you'll develop and remember your own favorites, your own sequences, your personal routine. But for the first run-through, I suggest you take this book to the floor with you, mark your place with your finger, and stretch, read, and stretch some more. And take your

---

*Ligaments are virtually unstretchable, in the sense of increasing their length, unless they're injured, i.e., partially ruptured. Healing may not restore their original length. You don't want to rupture your ligaments (or otherwise hurt yourself; see the rules, above). But a little gentle tension is another matter. You put a stretching force on the ligaments of your foot, for example, every time you take a step, and that tension helps maintain the ligaments' health. For a complete discussion of connective tissue, see chapter 5, "Connections."

time: try to make sure you've gotten all the good out of each
stretch before you go on to the next illustration.

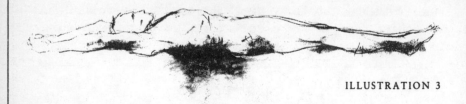

ILLUSTRATION 3

You've got to start somewhere: getting long and loose and
generally relaxed is as good a way to begin as any. Lie on your
back with your arms over your head, and stretch out as long as
you can. Simple as that.

But explore the possibilities of this simple stretch. First, relax:
get as flat to the mat as you possibly can. (If your shoulders or rib
cage are tight, you'll feel some stretching effect just from relaxing
with your arms over your head.) As you stiffen and straighten
your arms to reach upward, feel the stretch work its way from
your armpits down through your chest, your rib cage, your lower
back. (Start getting familiar with the sheets of fascia that envelop
your trunk.) With your legs still flat, curl your toes up toward
your head, pulling tight the calf muscles. Feel the stretch work up
the back of the knee. Then point your toes downward and clench
your buttocks, tilting your pelvis upward. (This is a good exercise
to help relieve sciatica-type pains in the buttock and back of the
leg.)

Relax, legs still flat, and bring one arm down to your side,
then reach upward hard with the arm that's still over your head,
pointing the toe of the leg on that side, paying particular attention
to the stretch of the area from armpit to thigh. You should find
yourself curving in an arc toward your relaxed side, pulling the
stretched side longer. Repeat with the other arm and leg.

Once I've got myself really flat on the mat, I like to bring my
knees up to my chest, curling into a ball, and rock slowly back
and forth, working the tissue along my spine.

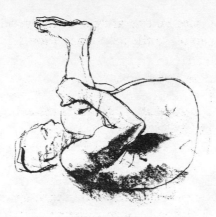

ILLUSTRATION 4

Gentle rocking works the vertebrae, getting them moving, opening up their joints for the flow of spinal and synovial fluids. (The spinal fluids have no circulatory pump: the only circulation they get comes from movement.)

As I rock, I hear some popping and cracking noises, signals that indicate a joint has moved and is therefore free to move again. That's why chiropractors crack your back. In the chiropractic view (as I understand it), many if not most of our musculoskeletal and neuromuscular ills develop out of the loss of mobility of the joints. Joints are to move. (Otherwise solid bone would do.) As aging tries to stiffen me, that viewpoint gets more convincing every day. Chiropractors have a lot of success treating athletic injuries.

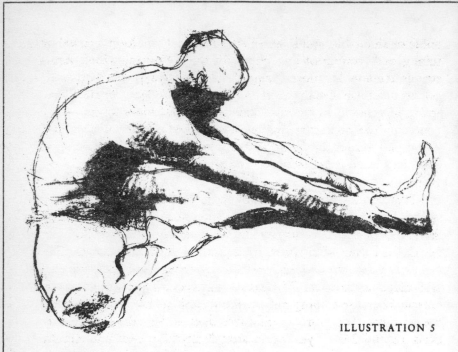

ILLUSTRATION 5

This is the basic hamstring stretch, the keystone of every stretching program, the most popular stretch of all. There are all kinds of ways to stretch your hamstrings; one of the most popular, standing with the foot up on a fence rail or wall, is also the riskiest: it's too difficult to maintain balance. Some track and field athletes and other ultrasupple jocks like to tuck a foot back to the outside and hyperflex the knee, making it into a hurdler's stretch: a very extreme position, hard to control, and on Dr. Dominguez's hit list. Fragile knee joints don't want a whole lot of stretching. I prefer the version illustrated here because of its triangulated stability, which makes relaxation so much easier, and because it gives you two extremely satisfying ways to go when you're ready to move on to new tissues.

The starting position is simple enough, and gets at a great deal of tissue that seems always to be ripe for stretching. Remember to relax your upper body (along with everything else you can possibly relax). If you can't comfortably reach your foot, grab your ankle or shin—but you'll have better results if you loop a towel or tubing over your foot and pull with that. Women, whose hamstrings tend to be more flexible, may have to reach farther to get an effective stretch. Start out by concentrating on the hamstring in general, but notice that if you bend more at the waist you can move that stretching tension up the back of your leg, and if you pull harder on your foot, you move the tension down your leg. The stretch is intensified if you gradually relax your neck and drop your head.

Try working the tension slowly up and down the leg a few times. There are real riches here. The hamstring is a group of three very large, very strong muscles between the butt and the back of the knee which provides much of our running power. The calf is a group of two large muscles—*gastrocnemius* and *soleus*—plus three small ones. The gastroc is predominantly fast-twitch muscle fiber for leaping and sprinting; the soleus is slow-twitch for stamina. (For more specific stretches of the calf, see illustrations 12 and 26.) If you never stretch anything else, you should stretch out your hamstrings and calves regularly: they are hard-used muscle groups, very susceptible to tightening and shortening, particularly from running—the most predominant athletic activity of all. As a result, the back of the leg—hamstrings, calf, Achilles tendon—causes athletes perhaps more trouble than even the lower back (which is also stretched by these same moves).

As you stretch, try twisting the foot of the straight leg from side to side, to move the tension from one side of the Achilles tendon and the lower calf to the other. Feel the extensive sheets of connective tissue that surround the ankle. Alternately point the toe—increasing the stretch on the shoulders and lower back—and raise it, increasing the stretch on the calf. Pull with the opposite arm (right arm when you're stretching left hamstring, and vice versa) and feel the connective tissue pull taut all the way down into the hip. Tighten one arm, then the other, varying the tension that's transferred to the trunk and lower back.

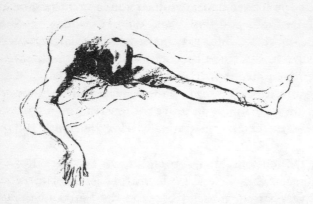

ILLUSTRATION 6

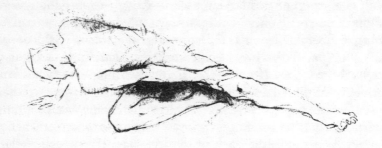

ILLUSTRATION 7

When you've run out of possibilities in illustration 5, let go with the arm opposite the straight leg, and brace that elbow on the bent knee. Slowly swing your head and shoulders down and forward, toward the bent knee, while pushing with your elbow. You'll stretch the groin of the extended leg and, simultaneously, the trunk on the opposite side. That's the first move from the hamstring stretch. There's a great deal of tissue to stretch as you move your upper body back and forth in a slow, relaxed arc between your knees.

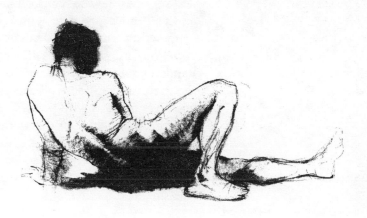

ILLUSTRATION 8

For the second move, go back to the starting position (illustration 5), then let go with your arms and roll your body over your straight leg, using the arm on the straight-leg side to brace yourself. The stretch moves to the hip and lower back. Your weight on your braced arm will also further stretch the shoulder on that side, the rib cage, the lower gut. (Just leaning on an elbow stretches the shoulder nicely, if you relax and let the weight be taken up in the joint capsule.) You may want to roll back and forth between the starting position and these two moves. When you're done, repeat with the other hamstring.

By now you'll notice a lot of repetition: these stretches keep returning to the lower back, the rib cage, the hips, and the groin. That's deliberate. You'll usually find it feels good to go back and stretch these areas again. Every new way of getting at them seems to stretch them a little differently, a little more productively.

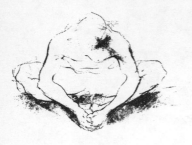

ILLUSTRATION 9

While you're sitting, here's a simple groin stretch. This position doesn't allow much movement, but it's very stable and controllable, and you can experiment with it to suit your own needs. You can push your knees downward with your hands or your elbows to increase the stretching tension; you can pull your feet upward with your hands to work the outside of the ankles. Try dropping your upper body forward—completely relaxed—and then swinging it in a slow arc from one side to the other.

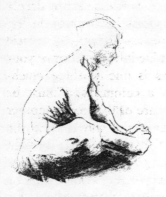

ILLUSTRATION 10

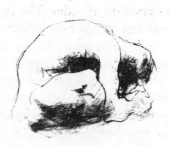

ILLUSTRATION 11

Lean your upper body forward with your head and shoulders erect, and the stretch concentrates in your lower back; drop your head and the stretch will emphasize neck, shoulders, and upper back. If these moves aren't sufficient, straighten your legs and spread them wide, then repeat the body lean through the available arc.

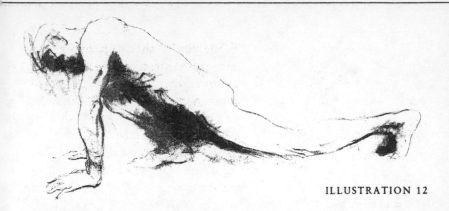

ILLUSTRATION 12

This is another deceptive stretch. It starts out stretching your hip, groin, and upper thigh, and then, as you ease more deeply into it, works its way around the lower gut and the rim of the hip bones. Most particularly it gets at the *psoas*—that tricky muscle group that ties the front of your lower spine into the front of your pelvis and the lower belly. The psoas is one of three much-neglected muscle groups. The spine is a column and must be guy-wired on all sides. The psoas takes care of the front; another group ties the lower rib cage and sides of the vertebrae to the pelvis; a third group holds the back side of the spine upright between the neck and the butt. These three groups stabilize the largest hinge in the body, the waist. They are not the sort of muscles that body-builders try to build up into bulging glory, not symbolic of power and strength like thighs and biceps, but upright human movement can't be launched without their elegant coordination and support. When we think we're in shape for just about anything, and then try some unaccustomed athletic activity, these are the muscle-tendon groups that complain the loudest, that get the sorest. The least we can do for them is to give them a good stretch now and then. Mine certainly appreciate it, anyway.

Keep your forward heel on the floor to reduce strain in the bent knee joint. If you drop your upper body low, alongside your bent knee, you'll stretch out the bent leg's hip and its extenders: the musculature of the butt, upper hamstring, and back of the thigh.

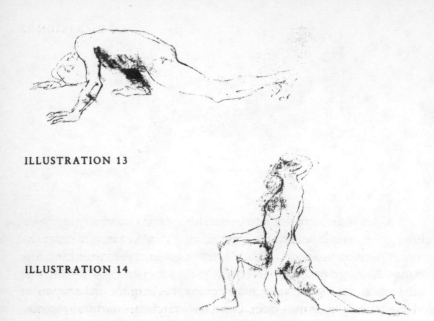

ILLUSTRATION 13

ILLUSTRATION 14

Pull your upper body upright, and the stretch moves to the hip flexors and front of the thigh on the straight-leg side. Keep your weight on the top of the foot of the straight leg, and you stretch ankle and upper foot nicely. Try it also up on that toe, with the foot flexed, as in illustration 13. Rock back and you stretch the arch of that foot; rock forward and you stretch the arch of the other foot, of your bent leg. Interestingly, when you flex the foot with the leg straight, the gastrocnemius is stretched—that's the overlying sprinting muscle of the calf. But if the foot is flexed with the knee bent, it's the underlying soleus that is stretched. Reverse legs and repeat the above moves, and you attend to both muscles in both calves.

Once you've thoroughly explored the possibilities of illustrations 12, 13, and 14, you can roll out of the position to the straight-leg side, supporting your weight with your arms, and move the stretch from the front of your body to the side. Now you're really getting at the rest of that girdle of tissue that is responsible for keeping you a biped.

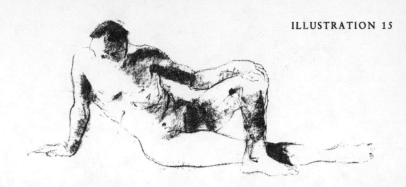

ILLUSTRATION 15

Pause there, explore the possibilities. Then switch legs. Pause also for a while with both legs straight behind you, hanging on your supporting arms. When you do, you're reconfirming the range of flexibility of your lower back, and giving the front side of your entire trunk a good stretch in the bargain. When you've done both sides, you've completed the circle around your center section.

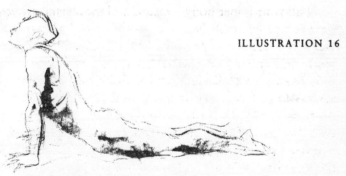

ILLUSTRATION 16

The next one gets two very different stretches out of one position. It's time to take care of the back side of the shoulder joints, as promised. (If you want to preserve the center-outward progression, this is a good place to insert the moves in illustrations 1 and 2.) The starting position looks more complicated than it is: sit comfortably crosslegged; raise one knee; lock the opposite elbow behind it.

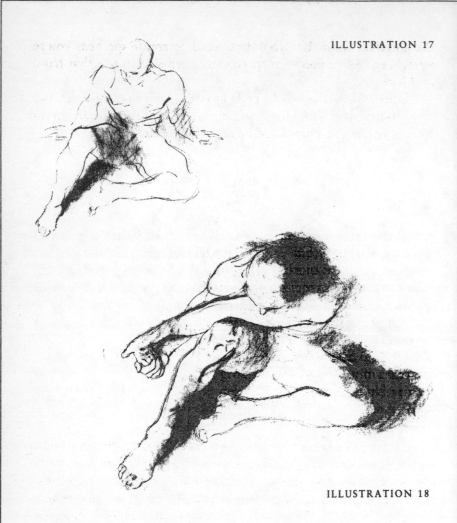

ILLUSTRATION 17

ILLUSTRATION 18

Rotate your shoulders toward the arm and hand that are pinned by your raised knee, and you stretch the back of that arm's shoulder joint—the part of the circumference of the shoulder joint that you couldn't really get at in the stretch in illustration 1. You'll want to spend some time gingerly feeling around in this position. If you back off tension and rotate the arm in its socket, you can work your stretch right around the back arc of the shoulder joint. Use your free hand to rotate the arm you're stretching. While you're at it, you can even stretch out that hand and forearm.

Once you've worked everything you can on that shoulder and arm, rotate your shoulders back in the other direction, and push against the raised knee with the arm you just stretched.

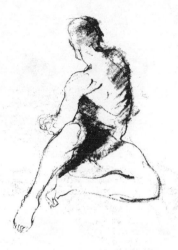

ILLUSTRATION 19

This is a powerful twist to the entire spine. By alternately curving and straightening the spine as you twist it, you can work the stretch up and down the back, in a virtual vertebra-by-vertebra progression. Ever eat the neck of a chicken? Picture that intricate structure. There's an enormous amount of connective tissue embedded within and around the spinal column: tiny muscles and their tendons that seldom get a thorough stretching out. As the discipline of yoga insists, the spine is the central skeletal fact—the locus of the life force. It deserves some tender loving care; other than rest on a good hard bed, gentle stretching is about all you can do for it.

The moves in illustrations 17, 18, and 19 need to be repeated for the other side, of course.

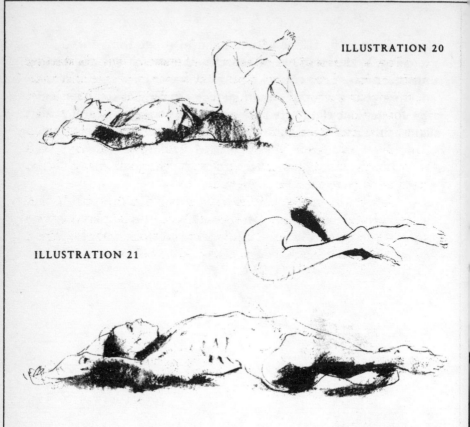

ILLUSTRATION 20

ILLUSTRATION 21

ILLUSTRATION 22

This is a clumsy-looking but extremely satisfying stretch. It gets at the psoas and just about everything else on the front side of the body above the knee. Lie on your back with your knees drawn up, hook one heel over the other knee, and press that knee to the floor. I lock my hands behind my head to start with, but when the pleasurable part of the stretching sensation begins to subside, I reach high with the arm on the side I'm stretching, which pulls tight everything from knee to armpit. No other stretch I know of lets you feel the extent of the fascial sheets so clearly. I usually do each side two or three times.

*   *   *

That's the last of the basic group of moves. These six starting positions have been chosen mostly for *length*: with the exception of those that work the vertebrae, they are designed to stretch out the longest muscles of the body, to work on the tissues that span and tie together the maximum lengths between attachment points. The longer the tissue, the more stretchability it will have, and therefore the more there is to work with. The goal, always, is the restoration of relaxed resting length.

After you've completed the basic group, you'll probably find a few details still to clear up—special needs, special parts of your anatomy that are used hard in the way you work and play. I'm a swimmer, so my shoulders can always use help.

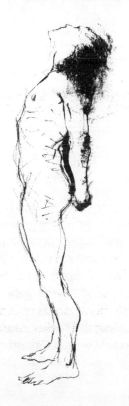

This is the essential swimmer's stretch. (I find myself doing it several times a day, anytime I feel tension building in my shoulders.) I start simply by clasping my hands behind my butt, arms straight, and pulling hard, pushing my breast up toward the ceiling.

ILLUSTRATION 23

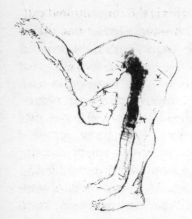

ILLUSTRATION 24

Then I bend at the waist and slowly let my arms sag as far over my head as they'll comfortably go.

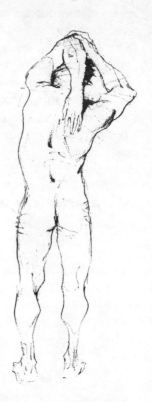

ILLUSTRATION 25

One more for the shoulders: this is the way most stretching manuals would have you stretch them out. Exert pressure against the bent elbow with your head. It isn't as good as the earlier stretches for exploring the entire range of motion of the shoulder, but it has the advantage of stretching the neck as well. You can push back with your head to increase tension against your arm; you can contract your arm and shoulder muscles to push against your head and stretch your relaxed neck. One hand washes the other.

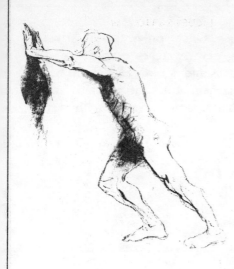

This is the conventional calf stretch—and another one that's easy to sneak into the middle of a busy day. Note that one leg is bent (stretching the soleus), the other straight (gastrocnemius). You can get at these muscles a little more specifically from this starting point than you do with illustrations 12, 13, and 14. As usual, I always find myself rolling my body from side to side, and sagging toward the wall as I do. This moves the stretch from the calf to the trunk and psoas.

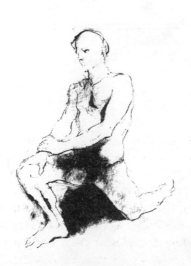

ILLUSTRATION 27

Another sneaky stretch. Anytime I can find an occasion to drop to one knee—beside my desk or anywhere else—I surreptitiously stretch out my psoas, groin, and hip flexors. From the illustrated starting position, you apply tension simply by pushing your hip forward and leaning back. The more arch you put in your back, the higher you move the stretch, from thigh right on up to upper rib cage. End up with your head back, and you stretch the front of your neck from chin to breastbone.

*　*　*

That ought to give you the idea. Once you've got the principle, you'll find yourself inventing new stretches everywhere, as
you lean against doorways, as you sit and read, even lying in bed.
(I have a chinning bar in my basement, for example, and have
grown to love simply hanging from it, stretching from elbow to
toe.)

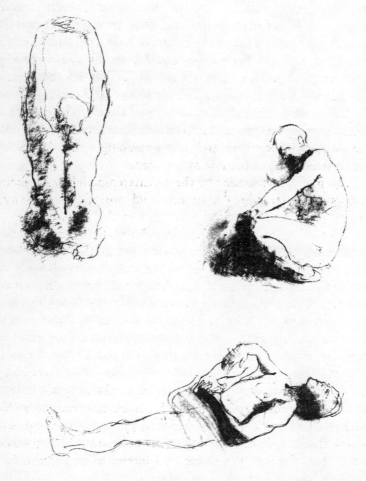

I must confess that I'm not certain I do these stretches in this order, in quite this way. I just get down on the mat and stretch what seems to need it, in the order in which it calls itself to my attention. I do try to take care of the large muscle groups every day, but I've gradually learned how to find and get at where I'm stiff, where I hurt—places I've missed with my regular routine. I go to those places and take care of them, and by the time I'm done I've pretty well covered the waterfront. For small muscle groups in unusual places—the kind that get tight and sore from unusual activities—I may have to invent new stretches, but I don't think of it that way any longer. I just work the joint in that part of its range of motion that allows me to feel the stiffness, and then figure a way to pull out the stiffness. There is no position in which you can't find a bit of purchase, a nice long muscle that wants drawing out, an undiscovered tightness that can be alleviated only by a long slow pull of lengthening tension. That's the way to stretch: by need, not by numbers.

You may be persuaded by the antistretching lobby to abandon programmatic stretching as a pre- and postathletic activity, as part of your fitness routine. Fine. But you're not going to stop stretching when you get up from your desk or when you get out of bed in the morning. I recommend you build on that—on that entirely natural impulse—rather than on dubious stretching-manual exercises (including, perhaps, the above) and their rigid forms and headlong pursuit of range of motion. You'll feel better for it.

One last word. I spoke earlier of stretching while watching TV. You can do that, although I'm sure it's a bad idea. (If I stretch to music it makes me *softer,* somehow, and I can find more to let go of within the muscle.) The thing about stretching is that you can do it very effectively without thinking about it, but you can do it a lot more effectively if you *do* think about it. While doing it. This isn't a cult of disciplined practices (although sometimes I think it ought to be). There are surely better ways to stretch than the way I'm doing it. I intend to find them. In the meantime, this is a good way to start.

PART II

THE PHYSIOLOGY OF SUPPLENESS

Anatomy may not be destiny, but it is all we bring into this world and all we can take away with us when leaving. Not that we are endowed at birth with a fixed and changeless structure; it is dying and being reborn continually. But in this intricate, dense, moist web of cells we carry around with us (and not in any airy thing attached to it) lies the substance of all the love and hate, joy and grief, hardheaded analysis and excited imagination we experience during our sojourn on this planet. And it is only because certain cells make signals, chemical and electrical, to communicate with each other, that we are able to think and feel at all.

Melvin Konner—*The Tangled Wing*

CONNECTIONS

Connective tissue is the stuff that weaves the body into one flexible piece; its ramifications for suppleness, and for hard use of the body, are therefore enormous. Muscle generates force, but connective tissue is the medium through which that force is turned into movement. In the simplest view, connective tissue is tendon, which connects muscle to bone, and ligament, which ties bones together. Clench a fist: the tendons that stand out on the inside of your wrist connect the muscle of your forearm to your hand and fingers, pulling on them to make them move. Rotate your wrist: ligaments set the limits to that motion.

Connective tissue, however, is much more than tendon and ligament. It is the webbing that holds our basic physiology together, the organizing principle of the body. It is the material that covers our body inside and out, lines the bones, contains the organs, delineates our internal boundaries. It is the structural material of the lungs and the diaphragm, and it forms the arterial walls. It constitutes the vast sheets of fascia that overlie the musculature and stabilize the major body elements, the sheaths that pull diverse muscle fibers into coherent units. Every muscle fiber has its own sheath of connective tissue; without it, muscle tissue would be nothing but stringy gelatin.

When you train, healthy connective tissue is the stuff that contains and accommodates your efforts, that binds into place the changes that training brings. When you injure yourself, what you hurt is more likely to be connective tissue than anything else, particularly if the injury is from inappropriate use: connective tissue is where both under- and overuse injuries strike first. Connective tissue is the missing link in the athletic equation. It's worth caring for.

Because the body is a single, flexible unit, forces working on connective tissue at any point transmit force everywhere else. A sore ankle changes loadings not only on the opposite hip but on that shoulder. Working effectively with this transmission of force is the key not only to successful training but to rehabilitating injuries and to maintaining suppleness. This is a reasonably simple principle, but its effects, in application, become very complex. Unfortunately, it's a concept that traditional athletic thinking—and traditional medicine—too frequently overlook.

At the simplest level, tendons carry the force generated in the muscle across the hinge of the joint to move the bone on the other side. But the transmission of force is seldom that simple, because few joints are that simple; most work through several planes of motion, operated by multiple muscle-tendon units. These muscle-tendon units work together simultaneously for large efforts, or in elaborate and delicate coordination for complex motions. The broader the joint's range of motion, the more different muscle groups will be needed to power it, supplying more angles of tension. Eleven major motor muscles (with tendons on each end) are needed to give the shoulder its range and accuracy—sufficient for everything from throwing 98-mile-per-hour fastballs to guiding hands through eye surgery.

During heavy efforts and complex motions, the work load is distributed among the muscle groups. When injury or fatigue strikes, the weakest, lightest, least responsive muscle in the group is the one that will fail first. Its failure forces other muscle-tendon units in the group to compensate, overloading them. When one muscle compensates for another, it works its connective tissues at new angles, out of their usual alignments, loading joint crossings and attachment points in unaccustomed directions. If you try to continue an athletic motion when muscles are beginning to fail, you'll modify your motion slightly, in search of a combination of muscles or an alignment that will reduce the pain but permit the motion to continue. You'll lift or drop your elbow, push off differently with your feet. A limp is nothing more than an attempt to continue an accustomed motion using uninjured tissues.

The modified motion, however, spreads the stress outward from the injured unit: tendon injuries have a way of begetting tendon injuries. Stress to connective tissue at any point spreads stress everywhere else. When muscles are held in tension over time, whether from physical or emotional pain, their connective tissue eventually shrinks to the contracted length, binding the shortness in place. Shortened muscles, like injured ones, also change the loading on surrounding connective tissue, which transmits the changes onward. The stress thereby imprints itself, uncannily, in the connective tissue.

This imprinting, storage, and transmission of trauma sounds a little too mystical for more conservative practitioners, who often dismiss it as subjective, imagined. But the mechanism for registering injury is clear, and follows the accepted principles of work physiology. Even a few days with a sore ankle, for example, will be recorded elsewhere at least semipermanently. When you limp to ease the load on that injured ankle, you favor one calf muscle while loading the other. The underloaded calf begins to atrophy from its reduced work load; the other calf, now overloaded in accordance with standard strength-training practice, begins to grow larger and stronger.

Compensating for the strength differential at the calf, you are forced to load thighs and hips differently: one side grows stronger with work, the other weaker with inactivity. The effect spreads to the muscles of the spine. When one side of the spine is strong and the other side weak, you change the way you generate and apply force in every direction. Working the weak side requires more energy, thereby increasing the load even to the heart, that infallible tachometer of effort.

Thus the effects spread from the sore ankle like ripples in a pond (and vice versa: a source of chronic ankle sprains is often a weak hip). The injury is gradually imprinted throughout the body, and traces of it remain after the injury site itself is healed. The traces can manifest themselves in anything from scar tissue to malformed bone, from reduced range of motion to changes in cardiac function. There's nothing mystical about it. The medium in which the traces are laid down, and through which the message is transmitted, is connective tissue. Scrupulously complete rehabilitation is required to balance out injured and uninjured body parts: merely resuming normal use will not correct the imbalance.

Injuries only dramatize this mechanism; forces are being transmitted throughout the connective tissue whether you are injured or not. It's the way the body works. If we understand the mechanism best through injury and rehabilitation, that's because connective tissue does get injured a lot. This shouldn't be surprising: where hard use is concerned, connective tissue is our weakest link.

That sore ankle, for example, would most likely be Achilles tendinitis—inflammation of the tendon that connects calf muscles to heel bone, one of the most common athletic injuries. (The legend of Achilles' heel springs from the vulnerability of that part of the anatomy, not because of its exposed location but because of troublesome mechanics in foot, heel, calf, and their juncture. It's a bad design.) Other forms of tendinitis, including tennis elbow and shin splints, vie with the Achilles for most frequent injury. I haven't seen the statistic collected, but the overall category of tendinitis is surely the most frequent class of sports injury. It is a connective tissue injury, of course.

Sprains and strains are also connective tissue injuries; "muscle" tears and pulls and charley horses are damage to the connective tissue that sheathes the muscle as much as to muscle fiber itself. Full use of the muscle isn't regained until its connective tissue heals. You can't injure muscle or bone without injuring the tissue that covers it, and the muscle and bone will heal more quickly, and almost surely more completely and satisfactorily, than the connective tissue will.

Among the nonathletic, most of the little "cricks" and "twinges" that unaccountably come and go are low-grade connective tissue injuries. (Without a fundamental level of suppleness, any sudden or forceful move can tear connective tissue.) Connective tissue problems can be the real culprit in back problems and in the skeletal changes associated with aging, in vascular disease, in loss of respiratory capacity and cardiac function, even in the creeping nearsightedness of middle age.

THE STUFF ITSELF

In our efforts to keep connective tissue supple, it's helpful to know what it's made of. All connective tissue is comprised of the same materials, wherever it is located in the body, whatever function it serves. The proportions of those materials and their physical arrangement vary to suit the specific anatomical requirement. The major structural components are two kinds of protein-based fiber and a ground substance. One fiber, *collagen*, provides tensile strength; the other, *elastin*, gives connective tissue its elasticity. The ground substance, a *mucopolysaccharide*, functions both as a lubricant, allowing the fibers to slide over one another with little friction, and as a kind of glue, holding the fibers of the tissue in a comprehensive mass. If you think of connective tissue as a kind of fiberglass that didn't harden, then collagen and elastin are the fiber, and the ground substance is the glass.

The trouble with connective tissue is that it deteriorates both from under- and overuse. With aging, and its attendant underuse, the fiberglass begins to set. The elastin frays and loses its elasticity, the collagen increases in stiffness and density; the tissue strengthens but also pulls ever tighter. That's why we shrink and fold in upon ourselves as we age. With overuse, on the other hand, the connective tissue begins to suffer something very like metal fatigue, the individual fibers wearing out and rupturing. Ruptured connective tissue heals, but slowly: orthopedists would much prefer to deal with fractured bone than torn tendon.

To understand how connective tissue functions in the real

world, tendinitis is a good starting place. The causes of chronic tendinitis are known (we think) and its prevention understood, but its cure—the unambiguous solution to the problem that we expect from modern medicine—continues to elude us. (Treatment, essentially, is rest, ice, and aspirin.)

"Tendinitis" simply means swelling of the tendon. You can get it from pruning roses or doing too much of anything else that requires a repetitive motion. It usually feels like a kind of internal rawness, with symptoms ranging from an occasional piercing sharpness at sudden movement to a dull ache at night. Although it may not always feel joint-related, it is, because tendons work across joints, as in the wrist. A joint is a corner, and a tendon is a cable that transmits force around corners. Tendinitis develops when the cable isn't flexible enough for its corner.

There is some sort of tendon on each end of every skeletal muscle, and there are at least six hundred skeletal muscles. If you envision the tiny muscles that align and stiffen the spine between each vertebra—each with its miniature tendons and attachment points—you begin to sense the complexity of the problem. All those spinal muscles and their associated connective tissues, by the way, need their own appropriate levels of activity, not only to maintain suppleness but to avoid the legendary miseries of the bad back.

The tendon itself is a bundle of microscopic fibers wrapped in a sheath, richly supplied with nerves but poorly supplied with blood, particularly at the junctions with bone and muscle. (The rich nerve supply speeds pain signals; the poor blood supply slows healing.) Tendinitis is always mechanical in origin, caused by structural breakdown from wear or trauma. When structural failure begins, the weakest fibers rupture, increasing the load and the risk to the remaining fibers—just as when one unit of a muscle group starts to fail. The ruptures cause the tendon to bleed or "weep"—exuding fluids much as when you stick a finger in your eye. (One folk name for a particular kind of tendinitis is "weeping sinew.") These fluids cause the inflammation that gives tendinitis its name; they also play a role in healing.

Once a weak spot is established in the tendon, continuing the load can make the failure progressive. Ballet dancers and serious athletes sometimes snap a tendon—usually the Achilles, allowing calf muscles to roll up like a window shade. Immediate surgery is required to repair the damage. Most of us seek relief before that occurs.

Relief is curiously hard to come by. Orthopedists traditionally lay out three not terribly encouraging treatment options: injection, surgery, physical therapy. Injection (usually a corticosteroid) treats the pain, not the injury, and weakens the tendon. It also requires an injection at every single injury site in order to be effective, and in complex structures such as the shoulder this is practically impossible. Surgery is indicated only for a limited range of tendon injuries, and sometimes doesn't work anyway. Physical therapy is the obvious conservative first choice.

Therapy may include ultrasound, gentle massage, stretching, anti-inflammatory medication, ice packs, and some very careful exercises in progressive overload: weightlifting, really, but starting with gentle, small movements, against resistance no greater than the weight of the affected limb. The exercises are refined, ultraspecific versions of the same movements that damaged the tendons in the first place. This may seem maddeningly illogical, but isn't; you rebuild strong tendons the same way you build or rebuild strong muscle and bone—with progressive overload. It is one kind of appropriate level of use.

These rehab exercises demonstrate the role of tension in maintaining the healthy connective tissue that suppleness requires. It's the collagen fibers that fail in tendinitis. Healing takes place in two stages. Strands of new collagen are first laid down in the injury site in random fashion—"like spaghetti in a bowl," as therapists are fond of saying. This disorganized collagen is scar tissue: only a patch, with little useful strength. In the second stage, the collagen begins to be remodeled into proper tendon. For that remodeling to take place, tension is necessary. The collagen fibers reorient themselves in line with tensile force applied to the tissue. Stretching the tendon—whether by working the muscle or performing stretching exercises—supplies the tensile force. Without it, the collagen remains mere scar tissue, and the resulting weak spot will virtually assure that the tendinitis becomes chronic.

The healing of connective tissue is further complicated by the chemistry of the injury cycle. The fluids that accumulate about the injury site contain enzymes that break down collagen, to help clean up broken bits of tissue. Inflammation actually kicks off the healing process in the first place, so it is necessary. If it goes on too long, however—beyond forty-eight hours or so—it starts to work against the formation of sound new collagen. Rehabilitative exercise severe enough to cause new swelling can be counterproductive. (Ice and aspirin help keep down this swelling and thereby protect the new collagen: they're not just to make you hurt less.)

Too little rehabilitative exercise is equally harmful. Without tension, new collagen not only is left disorganized, it is eventually reabsorbed by the system. There is a decrease in the tensile strength of the fibers. The collagen content of the connective tissue won't be fully restored until its fibers are aligned by work. Somewhere, then, between tension enough to align the new fibers and tension enough to rupture them is a mysterious window of healing. Successful rehabilitation must take place within that vague window. It is a window of appropriate use.

Rehabilitation and training are different names for the exact same process. Rehabilitation of injury is ultraspecific athletic training, with the principles of physiological increase and improvement applied directly to the specific weakness left by the injury.

Suppleness depends almost entirely on healthy connective tissue. Connective tissue, like the muscle tissue with which it functions, is kept healthy by regular loading at an appropriate level of intensity and frequency. That means that in addition to all that other good stuff that exercise can accomplish, it helps keep your connective tissue healthy.

Exercise alone, however, is not always thorough enough, is difficult to control precisely enough, and carries side effects—including the shortening of connective tissues. Exercise is not always possible or even congenial. Stretching—a more accurate (and pleasurable) way of working the connective tissues—always is. The key to staying supple is to provide the connective tissue with the stretching it needs. That's why you want to think about stretching connective tissue, more than muscles and joints, as you design your stretching program to fit your personal needs and dimensions.

MOTORS

When I sign my name I make an act of will, but my fingers move in response to a battery of little "engines": the wrist is steadied by another lot placed in the forearm; in turn the forearm is controlled by others in the upper arm, the upper arm by others in the shoulder, while the shoulder is made firm by bringing into play a battalion of "engines" which support the backbone. No wonder forgery is so difficult.

—John Stewart Collis, *Living with a Stranger*

The robot TV camera pans, swivels, zooms in on the action. It moves whenever its target does: the lens swings horizontally, pauses, adjusts vertically, locks on, screws itself into focus. Each separate movement brings the whir of small electric motors. Science fiction movies use this kind of eerie mechanical selectivity to create dread: our hero in the hands of the machine.

There shouldn't be anything dreadful about it; the human eye works the same way, without the hum. Without the *audible* hum of motors, anyway. Half a dozen small muscles attach (with tiny tendons) to the eyeball on one end, to the skull on the other. Muscles on each side give the eyeball horizontal movement, and on top and bottom give it vertical movement; two more muscles, attached at top and bottom but anchored at the side, rather than at the back, rotate it in its socket. (One of these actually anchors at the back, but its tendon runs through a bone loop in the eye socket, a pulley that transmits force around the corner at a 90-degree angle to its line of attachment.) Other muscles within the eye adjust for light by pulling on the iris to control the size of the pupil, and for focus by varying the thickness of the lens, and therefore its focal length. These are the eye's motors. The eye is a muscular, and very busy, place.

The robot's motors move the lens in one plane at a time, which is why one hum follows another; the eye muscles act in fine coordination to allow you to cut angles, roll your eyes, swing them in sweeping curves. Your eye muscles don't do anything that the robot's motors can't do, but they do it simultaneously instead of serially. By now modern robot technology very likely permits such simultaneous work, but the programming that would permit such coordinated action must be excruciatingly complex. Your brain writes this program for your eyes—and hard-wires it into place—in the first few months of life.

Muscle, in other words, is also a network. We think of our muscles too specifically, of biceps and hamstring and calf, when in the flow of real-life use those units never function in such isolation. The movement that muscle makes possible is too complex; we perform the simplest acts too inventively. If we seldom contract single, isolated muscles, we also can't stretch isolated muscles back out again, no matter how specifically most stretching programs describe the task. What we stretch are networks of connective tissue and muscle, inextricably intermixed. The ways they are injured and repaired are similar, and both can lose suppleness from hard use. But muscle, unlike connective tissue, has *efferent* nerve endings; it is the stuff that acts, that makes movement. And when we stretch, we stretch muscle as well as connective tissue, so the more we know about how it works, the more effectively we can keep it supple.

In pursuit of specificity, kinesiologists assign roles to the muscles used in any movement. The *agonist* is the principal mover; it may be augmented by other muscles, but it is the central power supply in making any given move: the biceps, for example, when you bend your arm. The *antagonist* is the muscle opposite the move, in this case the triceps. Antagonist becomes agonist when you reverse directions and straighten your arm again. A *stabilizer* is a muscle that steadies or supports the joint, or the bones on the other side of the joint, against the pull of the agonist. A *neutralizer* is a muscle that cancels out extra motion from the agonist. Many muscles can pull in two directions at once; the neutralizer ensures that the contraction works in the desired direction. There may be several stabilizers and neutralizers at work at any joint, in any movement.

Although muscles can only pull, they can exert a pulling force without actually shortening: "contraction" refers only to the generation of tension. Muscles may contract *concentrically,* shortening against the load, as when you lift a weight; *eccentrically,* lengthening as they resist the load, as when you lower a weight; or *isometrically,* generating force but not changing in length, as when you hold a weight in place. In eccentric contractions, the antagonists are the ones doing the work.

This division of labor is simple enough in concept but maddeningly complex in operation. Antagonist muscles, for instance, must relax, letting themselves be pulled longer, to allow the movement itself (reciprocal inhibition), and then often must quickly contract to brake the movement, protecting the joint from damage. In forceful movements such as pitching a baseball, it is often stopping the motion, rather than starting it, that injures tissue. Stopping is an eccentric contraction, and eccentric contraction loads the muscle more heavily than concentric contraction.

There are also two-joint muscles—or, in the fingers, multijoint muscles, working across the wrist as well as all the joints of the finger. When you rise from a crouch, the quadriceps contracts at one end (to straighten the knee) and relaxes at the other end (to allow the hip to extend); when you kick a ball, the same muscle contracts at both ends at once, flexing the hip and extending the lower leg. During furious athletic action, such muscles are constantly switching back and forth from contraction to relaxation, from generating movement to stopping it in its tracks, from serving as agonist to serving as antagonist. Some movements require small muscle-tendon units to rotate bone ends past anatomical obstructions in the joint, kicking in and out like the control thrusters on spacecraft. (That's why, for example, you can't swing your arm through its maximum range of motion without rotating it in its socket.) Human movement is very complex; a simple contraction of a single muscle isn't likely to occur outside the laboratory.

When one muscle goes out of commission, from fatigue or injury, we can often find another to substitute, from somewhere nearby in the network of muscle that surrounds each joint. With this substitute muscle we can accomplish the same desired movement, or something reasonably close to it. If you've ever had to drive a lot of screws with a screwdriver, think of how many different ways you invented for twisting that blade, as your driving arm and hand grew progressively more tired. More often we are not substituting entire muscles but changing the percentage of load shared between cooperating muscles—a slight change in the rhythm of our efforts letting some muscles rest while others take over for a while. It is difficult to run a mile as fast on a treadmill as on a track because the pace is too regular. You can't switch loads to get any rest.

When we bring in fresh muscles and let others rest, we change the loading on all the other muscles, on all the structures of the joint itself. The medium of transmission of these changes is connective tissue. We use all of the parts of the body simultaneously, not serially. That's because they're *not* parts: we're one piece.

THE FIRING PIN

When we search out a substitute muscle, what we find is not so much muscle as new motor units. A motor unit is one motor nerve and all the muscle fibers into which it branches. When we send the nerve a signal, it contracts its muscle fibers. In areas where fine control is required, such as the eye, one motor nerve may fire only four or five muscle fibers; in muscles of gross movement such as the thigh, one motor nerve may fire a couple of hundred. When a muscle begins to fail, it is because it is running out of viable motor units. To keep going, you must somehow find and "recruit" more viable motor units.

How we find them is one of physiology's sweeter mysteries. We somehow search through our volitional capacity to find and fire just the right motor units that will best substitute for the ones that are going out of commission. There are plenty of motor units to choose from: we are oversupplied, and no one can fire more than a fraction of the available motor units of a given muscle at any one time. When the tiny woman lifts the car to free her child, it is because the adrenaline released in reaction to the emergency not only lets her generate more energy but helps focus her mind, enabling her to recruit more motor units. Some version of this same sort of focus—of access to motor units—is what allows one athlete to dominate his or her physical equal. The great athlete is better at recruiting motor units (among other things) than the merely good athlete. When an athlete reaches down for a little something extra—in strength or speed or endurance or even fine control—what he or she is reaching down *for* is more motor units.

The motor nerve and its muscle fibers constitute the essential athletic unit of power. Not surprisingly, a great deal of training is devoted directly to motor units. We train to prepare the accustomed motor units and their muscle fibers to function more quickly or strongly or to last longer before wearing out. We also train to accustom more motor units to the task. We used to think that the motor unit was either on or off, that it fired all its muscle fibers or none. Now we've determined that some muscle fibers have lower thresholds of excitability than others. So we train to improve the accessibility of the muscle fibers to voluntary control. Training reduces the strength of signal needed to fire a given motor unit. We train to learn *how* to reach down for a little more.

Viable motor units are the currency of muscular effort; once spent—with fatigue—they shut down, temporarily unavailable for work. A well-trained athlete has great wealth in available motor units, and the effectiveness of his or her performance depends almost entirely on how judiciously and appropriately those riches are spent. If you can manage to run out of motor units at the same time as you finish the contest, you've literally done the best you can.

When you do run out, what you've actually run out of is the capacity to fire the motor units. (A muscle that has been worked to failure, that you can no longer contract at all, will still contract in response to an electric shock.) You lose the capacity to fire the motor unit when too many of its muscle fibers signal the central nervous system that they are injured, or depleted of energy supplies and overloaded with waste products. These are the specific deficits that stretching addresses: gentle stretching of the muscle tissue hastens the healing of injured tissue, the replenishment of its energy, and the removal of wastes.

THE ARCHITECTURE

We are fibrous creatures, achieving movement only by tugging at our own strings. Just as our connective tissue is made up of threads, organized according to the direction of the pull, the muscle that does the pulling is also composed of fibers, arranged in bundles within bundles. The whole individual muscle—the biceps, for example—is enclosed in a bag of fascia. Within it are groups of bundles of muscle fibers, groups with their own separate sheaths, the bundles within individually ensheathed, the fibers themselves ensheathed yet again: layers upon layers of fibrous sheath. Within the smallest bundle is the individual muscle fiber, made up of thousands of *myofibrils*—the microscopic strings of protein that do the actual contracting. Strings within strings.

Attempting to apprehend muscle, science screws the electron microscope ever closer. At the microfibril level, the strands of protein are of two types, *actin* and *myosin*, lying alongside each other, making the muscle contract by crawling along each other's length. This interdigitation is powered by the formation and reformation of actomyosin cross-bridges, which lie along the length of the strands like teeth in a zipper. Burning energy makes a chemical change that causes the cross-bridges to break contact, flip forward, and reattach, ratcheting themselves along by molecular attraction. We move by swapping electrons at the molecular level: muscle turns chemistry into physics.

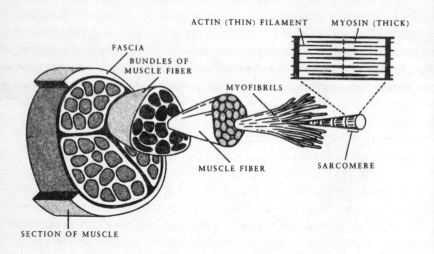

Although we think this is what happens, the action takes place on a scale too small to be observable. Some scientists believe that discovering what really goes on at the level of the actin and myosin fibrils is as crucial for the understanding of life as discovery of the structure of the atom was to understanding matter. Scientific cleverness hasn't yet been able to tease out the proof.

Cross-bridges aren't the only mystery: muscle is difficult stuff to study. I once asked exercise scientist Dave Costill, director of the Human Performance Lab at Ball State University, what a cramp is. "I'm glad you asked," he said, laughing in self-mockery. "We don't know. How're we going to study it? Dissect it while it's cramped?" We also don't know how muscle tissue grows larger and stronger (*hypertrophy*), although we know very well that it will do so if we load it progressively. For years we thought the individual fibers simply grew larger, and that you were born with your personal number of muscle fibers predetermined. Recently researchers have uncovered some division of fibers during hypertrophy, increasing their number. The research, using cats, requires counting the number of fibers at each end of a living muscle, causing it to hypertrophy by progressive overload (getting the cat to lift weights), and then recounting the fibers. Muscle is difficult stuff to study.

Still, we do know a little about it. Muscle is extensible and elastic: it can be stretched like an elastic band and will return to normal length. (So will tendon, but muscle tissue can be stretched to half again its resting length, tendon by only about 4 percent.) Muscle tissue is also capable of contracting to about half its resting length. The difference between maximum length and maximum contraction is the *amplitude of action*, which is what governs the active (as opposed to passive) range of motion.

If you stretch the muscle slightly just before contracting it, as in a backswing or wind-up, you can generate more power with it. Part of the gain is from increasing the distance through which force can be applied, but gain also comes from taking up the elastic elements of the muscle and tendon. When you start a movement with the muscle in an unstretched state, some of its contractile capacity—its amplitude of action—is used not to generate power but to take up the elasticity. If you start with the muscle under a slight stretch, as in a backswing, the stretch takes up the elasticity, and the muscle's entire capacity for contraction is available for powering the move. Stretching out the muscle first ensures that it has a chance to contract through the length at which it can produce the most power.

IMPLICATIONS

Stretching the muscle before contraction to gain power is sometimes mistakenly referred to as a stretch reflex. It isn't the stretch reflex (which is the knee-jerk response, the reflexive contraction of a muscle in response to a stretch from an outside agency), and it also doesn't have anything to do with programmatic stretching to maintain suppleness, no matter how stretching literature has strained to make the connection. Shortened muscles do generate less force, and muscles do shorten from either disuse or hard training. Stretching is a way of resisting that shortening and keeping it from becoming permanent. But that somewhat backward connection is the only direct one between stretching a muscle to generate more force and stretching a muscle to maintain suppleness.

There are subtler implications for suppleness, however, in the matter of the elastic components of the muscle-tendon unit. When scientists investigate mechanical problems involving muscle, they speak of the muscle's *spring stiffness*. Think of pulling on the ends of a coil spring; spring stiffness is the quality that resists stretching, that increases with the distance stretched. A muscle's spring stiffness is the sum of its elastic components and its contractile strength.

We usually perform our movements well inside the elastic limits of our musculature. Increasing those limits will increase the range of safe effort and therefore improve performance. Strength-building exercises improve the contractile component; stretching exercises improve the elastic component. You can generate more force in moves that pull the muscle out to length (yielding work, eccentric contractions) than you can in moves that shorten the muscle (gaining work, concentric contractions). Muscle-builders sometimes lower weights, rather than lift them, because eccentric contractions load the muscle tissue more heavily than concentric contractions and therefore build new muscle faster. Eccentric contractions also load the connective tissue more heavily, which may be why they make you sorer: hiking downhill hurts worse the next day than hiking uphill. Eccentric contractions take up the elastic components more effectively than concentric ones, but they tend to leave you working closer to the limits of safe effort, increasing the risk of damage.

Think of stretching as a kind of passive eccentric contraction, a way of helping maintain the elasticity of muscle and connective tissue without overloading it. Stretching, however, because it *is* passive, doesn't make you sore.

THE STRETCH ITSELF

There's another theory to explain the gain in force from stretching out the muscle to its best operating length. Under the microscope, skeletal muscle is striped, with alternating light and dark bands across the width of the muscle. The dark bands mark the areas of overlap of actin and myosin fibrils. Stretch the muscle too tight and the amount of overlap is reduced, so the fibrils get less purchase when they start contracting. But if you don't stretch it at all, the contraction may be started with the muscle already partially shortened, the overlap too great: there's less length for the actin and myosin to take up, and less force can be generated.

The stretching of muscle tissue takes place at the level of the *sarcomere*, which is also the essential unit of contraction in the muscle fiber. When the sarcomere contracts, the area of overlap of actin and myosin fibers increases; when the sarcomere is stretched back out, that area of overlap is reduced again.

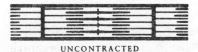

UNCONTRACTED

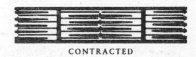

CONTRACTED

When the sarcomere is at its maximum resting length, the force required to lengthen it farther rises sharply. Additional lengthening force is taken up by the surrounding connective tissue; its collagen fibers are mostly slack until this rise in resting tension occurs, and then they begin to align with the tension. Thus when you stretch, you first pull the muscle out to optimum length for future action, sarcomere by sarcomere, and then, with further tension, you take the slack out of the connective tissue. When you do, you help realign any disorganized fibers with the direction of tension. That's the process that starts turning scar tissue into healthy connective tissue.

Muscle tissue is caused to contract by a signal like the ringing of a bell. It stays contracted as long as the signal goes on; when the signal stops, it is left adrift. The physical state of the fibers and the chemical products of contraction (and fatigue) are left essentially in place, unresolved. The impulse to stretch is the impulse toward resolution of the muscle's contracted state.

We think of relaxation as the opposite of contraction, but relaxation is nothing like that, it's just an absence of stimuli. Relaxation in the muscular sense accomplishes very little in the way of restoration, of preparation for future action. (Rest is not recreation.) Gentle movement, as in the cool-down, helps restore the musculature to suppleness and a ready state, since contraction of one muscle effectively stretches the others. But stretching is the important part. You want closure, completion, the function of the muscle taken through its full range of possibility. Stretching is the uncompleted half of every muscular contraction.

A PSEUDOSCIENTIFIC FOOTNOTE

What follows is a technical sidebar, intended for readers who are passionately interested in muscle. Skipping it won't seriously detract from your future stretching pleasures.

I've been trying for fifteen years or so to find out what goes on, mechanically, in muscle and connective tissue when you stretch it. There's no demonstrated need for this knowledge—I never supposed it would help me stretch better—but my way of grasping things is mostly visual, and without a mental picture I have trouble thinking about this or any other subject.

Circumstances bring me in contact with scientists in various fields, physiological and otherwise, and I never fail to ask them for hints or leads into the mechanics of stretched tissue. I've run into a striking lack of information about the subject. One friend who works in another area tells me that over the years he has passed my inquiry on to perhaps half a dozen specialists in muscle physiology. He too has continued to draw a blank. There is a peculiar scientific reticence about describing what takes place in soft tissue under tension.

The problem with the question is that it points to one of the more baffling mysteries about the stuff that powers every movement of every living member of the animal kingdom. For generations now, we've had this model of the basic structure of the muscle fiber, right there in the freshman physiology texts, but there's something about it that doesn't add up. Stretching, strangely enough, is part of that something.

Contraction occurs when energy is burned and the thin actin strands and the thick myosin strands crawl alongside each other, ratcheting the muscle fiber shorter. This is the "two protein" model, well established as current theory.

When you stretch relaxed muscle fiber, it resists—like a rubber band—with passive tension. The mystery has to do with the passive tension. When you pull on that relaxed muscle fiber, what is it you are actually pulling on? It isn't the actin fibers, which are physically connected only at the Z line of the sarcomere, not at the other end. And it isn't the myosin fibers, which are not connected structurally at *either* end. And it isn't the cross-bridges, which, in relaxation, we assume are disconnected.

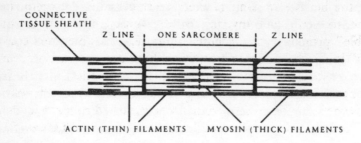

Obviously, what you're pulling on is the connective tissue—the sheath of collagenous fibers that encloses and supports the muscle fiber. Has to be. And in fact that's the interpretation espoused by modern exercise physiology. But there are indications that connective tissue, at least as we now understand it, doesn't quite explain the passive tension of muscle fiber. Researchers have managed to strip muscle fibers of their connective tissue sheath. These "skinned" fibers still show resistance to stretching. There seems to be something else besides actin and myosin fibers that ties the muscle fiber together. Unfortunately, the cleverest work so far has not succeeded in demonstrating what this something else is.

This is work that goes on at the level of electron microscopy, an attempt to unravel (literally) strands of protein so small and so fragile that they are more or less destroyed by any known method of dissection. Skinning them of their connective tissue is a remarkable technical feat in itself. It has even been proposed that actin and myosin themselves are artifacts of preparation, that muscle is actually a fiberless gel that somehow self-organizes under strain. Nevertheless, the actin and myosin structures have been accepted for decades. Nothing else has turned up with sufficient replicability to be accepted as scientifically proven.

So—assuming that the fibers are in fact skinned of their connective tissue—we have passive tension with no known source. Not too surprisingly, this has led to development of a heretical wing in muscle theory. The establishment holds to the two-protein model; the heretics are saying there must be a third protein, in addition to actin and myosin, in the muscle fiber. It is an "invisible" protein in one scientist's phrase, a "filamentous connection" in another's. Something like it has been demonstrated in insect flight muscle, a filament that connects the end of the thick filament to the sarcomere. It would be the missing thread that ties the sarcomere into a cohesive unit irrespective of connective tissue. It would be what you are pulling on when you stretch muscle tissue.

How many muscle proteins can dance on the head of a pin? The number of different kinds of protein in a muscle fiber, wherever they are attached, can hardly be critical to a successful and enjoyable stretching program. But I find a certain whimsical appropriateness to this mystery, given the controversy about the practice of stretching. The limits of scientific orthodoxy give us an incomplete picture. Nobody seems to *know* what you're pulling on when you stretch muscle tissue.

I believe the researchers will eventually demonstrate a third protein—or something else—that ties the sarcomere together structurally, with or without the connective tissue sheath. It won't be contractile, it'll be connective. (One suggested name for such a substance is *connectin*.) It will be another, different kind of connective tissue, surely elastic in nature. It will hold the contractile mechanism in place, aligned, organized, coherent. It will be the springy core at the heart of the muscle structure, the substance that gives muscle its supreme liveliness. But that is only my own unscientific conjecture.

In any event, muscle fiber suddenly becomes a much more complex place than we ever dreamed. Attempts to penetrate its mystery describe "core filaments," "side struts," "radial cross links," "elastic stroma." To the extent that any of these structures can be seen (by electron microscope), they seem to have a certain waviness not unlike the crimp in the threads from which stretch fabrics are woven. All of these proposed interconnections have a certain slack in one direction or another. Pulling on them pulls out the slack, organizes them into coherence.

Whatever the third protein is, in all its microscopic mystery, stretching it will do it a world of good, I'm sure of that. Contracting muscles keeps them alive, stretching them keeps them elastic. Keeps them, and thus you, supple. Function is maintained by use.

I can't imagine the structure of this substance, can't come up with a visual image of how it actually stretches or what stretching might do for it, but I find the notion positively charming: that there is some springy, elastic stuff at the heart of the muscle that is to all intents and purposes unknowable, and that in the end is what makes us *quick*—in the Shakespearean sense of the word.

Not science, not proved, but that's okay: it's something else to think about while I'm stretching. It's an entirely satisfactory way to understand what I'm feeling. If it's wrong, that's okay too: it'll do until new science comes along and gives me a better set of pictures.

INFORMATION

Muscle gets a bum rap. We speak of it as the opposite of brains, a metaphor for brute force and insensitivity. But no thought can be acted upon or any pleasure enjoyed without its help: we can't eat, drink, breathe, make love, work or play, take part in life—or maintain it—without muscle. We credit nerves for bringing us sensory richness, but without muscle to locate and process stimuli, those nerves would have precious little to work on. (Most sensors lose sensitivity quickly to a constant stimulus. We use movement to keep the stimuli varied. The movement comes from muscle.) Besides, living muscle is among the loveliest substances on earth to look at, to touch, and above all to use.

Furthermore, it's not dumb, not at all: it has its own remarkable intelligence-gathering capacity. If we don't learn to use and trust this intelligence, not only do we fail to get good use out of our muscle, but it's likely to start giving us trouble.

Muscle's intelligence-gathering capacity is a product of its dual function, which we almost entirely overlook. We think of muscle as the stuff with which we do things, but it is also the stuff that tells us what is done to us, what we've done to ourselves. Nerves run from the muscle as well as to it: it is as much a sensor as it is an effector. It senses a great deal. It reads the pull of gravity as surely as does the inner ear. It registers acceleration, deceleration, or any other change in physical loading. It tells us where we are in relation to the world, where our body parts are in relation to one another, how much force is needed for the next move in any direction. The musculature is a suit of power draped over our otherwise helpless bones, but it is also a suit of sensitivity, assessing our state and our situation, helping us respond more accurately to the world's requirements. Maintaining suppleness maintains that sensitivity.

Muscle's capacity for delivering information was driven home to me vividly late one night in a rear seat on a commercial aircraft. Looking up the long aisle, I watched the airplane change attitude, its nose lifting and dropping, swinging from left to right and back again. Then I realized I was seeing nothing of the sort: with total darkness outside, I could see nothing change its position in relation to anything else. There wasn't any movement to see. I was notified of the airplane's changes in attitude in small part by the balance mechanism of my inner ear and the skin of my backside, but mostly by my musculature, feeling gravity and momentum tug at my body mass from new angles. My brain translated what I felt into visual changes. I'd have sworn I was seeing it happen.

As a sensor, muscle is merely working with a different branch of physics from the more dominant eye. Interpreting light rays is almost algebraic, muscle sensing more geometrical—concrete, elementary, all forces and angles—but in the end both are electrochemistry. The various nerve endings may be fired mechanically, chemically, by heat or light, but the result of their firing is essentially the same: a signal to the brain. The brain turns the signal into sight, sound, sensation: information.

We do relish the swirl of information. Cultural evolution is a search for more and more sophisticated ways of firing off those sensory neurons; all our arts and leisures are the products of that search. Firing off the sensory neurons of our musculature—making fuller use of that huge sensory organ that is the one-piece body—is a terrific pleasure. We call it play or, in its more organized form, athletics.

THE OTHER SENSE

The nerve endings that pick up all that information from the musculature are the *proprioceptors*—"self-sensors"—which play an extraordinarily large role in athletics. They are *mechanoreceptors*, cranked into activity by actual physical displacement (movement) or would-be displacement (force). That's why they are of particular interest to anyone who would stay supple. They are worked—trained, improved, refined—by the same processes as those by which suppleness is maintained.

They constitute the most complex and elegant part of the physiology of movement. Physical skills—dexterity, timing, balance, accuracy, delicacy of touch, smoothness, reaction time, all those mysterious qualities that make up "coordination"—are largely a function of proprioception. The better the proprioception—literally the more, and more acute, the proprioceptive nerve endings—the better the athlete (or the performing artist). The more supple the musculoskeletal system, the more acute the proprioception.

The proprioceptors are nerve endings located in the joints, tendons, and muscles. They read the state and position of body parts, and any changes to that state and position, whether those changes are in loading, direction, or rate. The information they gather goes to both conscious and unconscious levels of the central nervous system: at the conscious level it informs our volitional actions; at the unconscious level it initiates and controls our muscular reflexes.

The proprioceptors in the joints are fired by pressure. There are two types. One of them, called the *Pacinian corpuscle*, reads pressures, but only briefly, accommodating quickly. This suits it well for picking up rapid changes but poorly for detecting constant pressure. When you run, these are the nerve endings that tell you where your feet are and how they should proceed: how much force from which muscles you're going to need next. The other type of joint receptor, the *Ruffini ending,* signals constant pressure, making it suitable for sensing joint position without movement. Each Ruffini ending monitors a specific portion of the arc of motion of the joint; the brain knows the address of each, and thus the joint's position.

When swelling changes the pressures within the joint, the readings from the joint receptors are affected. This can be disorienting. After extensive knee surgery, patients sometimes not only can't tell without looking what position their leg is in, but become so dissociated from it that they come to regard it as a foreign object in the bed with them. Other proprioceptors help read position sense, and will eventually take over for permanently damaged joint receptors.

The proprioceptors that are located in the tendons, called *Golgi tendon organs,* are fired by stretching. They have historically been regarded as a protective device, signaling excessive load. When a muscle begins to pull too hard on its tendon, the Golgi tendon organ signals the central nervous system to relieve the tension. An inhibitory reflex is fired, stopping the muscle's contraction. The muscle abruptly lets go, in the "clasp-knife response," to avoid injury. The sudden victory in arm wrestling comes when the loser's Golgi tendon organs kick in. It does so not by sending sensory information but by shutting down the muscle: you don't feel much of anything, you just collapse. When you're learning a new athletic motion, a proper follow-through is difficult: unfamiliar muscle tension fires the tendon organs' protective response, stopping contraction, ending the motion prematurely. You have to *learn* a new move—"groove" it—before you can put much force into it. Maximal strength depends in part on one's capacity to overpower the protectiveness of the tendon organs.

Injury prevention is a somewhat passive function of the tendon organ; recently we've learned that these sensors also take a more active role in proprioception, supplying the central nervous system with a continuous reading of the tension on the tendon—a filtered sample, in one researcher's description, of the active force being produced in the muscle. Tendon organs are in effect two-threshold organs. The lower threshold, which reads degree of contraction rather than likelihood of injury, is the organ's preferred level of stimulus.

Training lowers the active threshold and raises the passive one. That is, training increases sensitivity—the amount of information you get from the tendon organs—and at the same time raises the point of tension required for the muscle's collapse. You train any organ by using it, repeatedly taking it through its function. Tendon organs are stretch receptors; to train them, you work them, by stretching as well as by contraction. When you stretch them, they tell you how hard you are stretching and how hard you can safely stretch.

THE PHYSIOLOGY OF SKILL

The proprioceptors in the joints and tendons are relatively straight-forward; the proprioceptor in muscle, called the *muscle spindle,* is much more intricate in structure and in function than the other two. It too is a stretch receptor, but in this case is an almost Rube-Goldbergian neuromuscular feedback mechanism that not only tells us what our muscles are up to but actively contributes to the smoothness and control with which we use them.

The muscle spindle is a small bag of ordinary skeletal muscle fibers, inside which is a bundle of specialized muscle fibers. Picture an elastic cord inside an elastic bag, both capable of being stretched, both capable—separately—of contracting. The cord inside the bag, however, can contract only at its ends, not in its center. Contracting the ends stretches the noncontractile center section, which fires nerves that inform the central nervous system of the muscle's length, of any change in its length, and even of the rate of change of length.

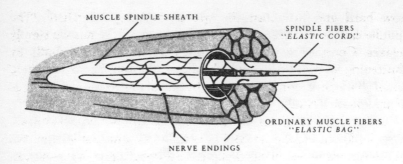

MUSCLE SPINDLE SHEATH

SPINDLE FIBERS
"ELASTIC CORD"

ORDINARY MUSCLE FIBERS
"ELASTIC BAG"

NERVE ENDINGS

MUSCLE SPINDLE

Such complex messages can be delivered because the bag and the cord inside it operate as a mutual feedback system. It is a servomechanism with two controls: the length and state of tension of the surrounding muscle fiber—the bag—and the length and state of tension of the cord, controlled by its own contractile capacity. This contractile capacity is the key to the spindle's multitude of functions. Because it can contract itself, and can compare its own tension to that of the surrounding muscle, the spindle stays fully operative no matter how the muscle changes length.

Among those functions is the stretch reflex: the tap on the patellar tendon pulls on the thigh muscle, which stretches the bag of fibers that is the muscle spindle. Stretching the bag stretches the cord inside, firing its nerve. That signal asks the central nervous system to contract the muscle in which the spindle is located; the knee jerks. Contracting the muscle shortens it, which reduces tension on the spindle, which turns down the signal.

What makes the spindle so complex is the cord's capacity to contract and stretch itself, on signal from the central nervous system. This allows it to continue to take readings, so to speak, whether the muscle is in action or not. But whether the source of the stretch is an internal command or an external force, the mechanical deformation sends a message back to the spine telling how hard and how fast the spindle is being stretched. (The spindle can also be stimulated in a third way: if the muscle simply relaxes. Contraction takes the stretch off the muscle spindle by shortening it; relaxation, which allows the muscle to lengthen, puts it back on again. Confusing, but invaluable for fine readings of the muscle's state.)

All this switching on and off of signals and of muscle contractions implies a certain amount of oscillation, and that's what we get. We learn to use it productively. *Postural sway,* for instance, enlists the stretch reflex to keep us upright. Sway in one direction and you stretch the muscles on the opposite side, firing their spindles, contracting them to pull the body weight back into balance. This oscillation spreads the work around among the antigravity muscles, allowing them occasional rest.

Standing is harder than moving, says Moshe Feldenkrais. Computers are being used to stimulate the leg muscles of paraplegics, helping them achieve a rudimentary form of walking. To enable the paraplegic simply to stand in place, however, an additional device, called the LSU brace, is required. Electronic pressure-receptors in the soles of the subject's shoes send signals to the skin of the chest, above the spinal lesion. The subject learns to read those signals with the skin of the chest instead of the feet, and, through a computer, to fire the muscles necessary to maintain balance. The LSU brace is, in other words, a computer-assisted, externally fitted stretch reflex.

Standing still is complicated; dynamically changing situations are no piece of cake either. Hold a book comfortably in your outstretched palm, elbow bent. Have someone drop an additional book onto the load. Your hand dips; this fires the stretch reflex in the biceps, causing you to contract the muscle, accelerating the hand and the books upward—usually too far. Contracting the muscle takes the stretch off the spindle, quieting its signal, telling you to diminish the contraction—usually too much, dipping your hand again, repeating the cycle on a smaller scale. Eventually you stabilize, the central nervous system somehow deciding how many motor units you need to steady the weight.

The more slowly the load is applied, the smaller the oscillation. The stronger reaction to sudden loading demonstrates the spindle's capacity to read rate of change as well as change itself. Where fine discrimination is required of the muscle, the supply of muscle spindles is richer. You have more muscle spindles in your thumb than in your thigh. (If you threaded needles with your knees, the distribution of spindles would be more equitable.)

This simplistic demonstration only hints at the intricacy of the muscle spindle's operation. Without looking, move your hand through a slow, smooth figure 8 in the air. The spindle's sensitivity to muscle length is what lets you know that you are making that figure 8; it is its sensitivity to rate of change that lets you know that you are making the move so slowly. It also helps you smooth out the sequence of muscle contractions. The muscle spindle is the device that allows you to make that motion in such stately fashion in the first place. It is the means by which you can give any characteristic you choose to any move you make. It can do so because it is sensitive to stretch.

The loop of nerves that maintains the muscle spindle's sensitivity is the *gamma system*. It ties the spindle's capacity to read change to its capacity to make change happen. If you are alive and neuromuscularly intact, you're sending a constant signal over the gamma loop: *to* the spindle to stretch the cord; *from* the spindle, describing that stretch. These signals continuously reset the muscle spindle with new information about the muscle's length—information that allows you to control style of movement.

Style of movement can be *phasic*—abrupt, sudden—in which case the motor nerves fire in waves; or can be *tonic*—slow and carefully controlled, the nerves firing continuously but asynchronously. The knee-jerk reflex is phasic, the postural reflex—that keeps you standing upright—is tonic. Tonic movements are more difficult (and more interesting) than phasic movements. At old-time fiddlers' contests, notice how the performances lose their precision in the slow parts: fast fiddling is easier than slow fiddling. Tonic movements require more skill. The muscle spindle is a phase damper, smoothing the waves out of the nerve impulses, turning phase into tone.

Tonic movements are possible only if the muscle is informed, in contact with itself. The contact is maintained, the muscle kept at the ready—cocked, in effect—by a low level of contraction on signal from the gamma system. That low-grade tension is *muscle tone;* it is palpable, even visible, in living muscle. Snip the gamma loop at any point and the tone is gone: the muscle goes flaccid and begins to atrophy. Nerve impulses are as necessary as oxygen and nutrients for the life of the muscle. Keep the signal turned on and muscle tone takes up the muscle's slack, keeping it purring away at idle, ready to respond without stumbling or lurching into motion. Without going phasic on you at the wrong time.

Muscle tone spreads its effects into our emotional lives. The gamma loop passes near the hypothalamus, the mysterious gland involved, according to the anatomy professor's old joke, in the four Fs—fighting, feeding, fleeing, and mating. The hypothalamus is also linked—we're not sure how—with our emotional state: electrical stimulation of the hypothalamus produces responses ranging from serenity to anxiety and terror. By some mechanism that also is not entirely clear, hypothalamic activity increases gamma system activity.

This is how mood is connected to posture. Upbeat emotional states—happiness, alertness, attentiveness—are reflected in increased muscle tone, upright posture, a kind of quick and bright physical approach to the world. We slump and sag from depression and unhappiness as dramatically as we do from fatigue. This isn't the "body language" of pop psychology, it's physiology, laid right down in muscle and nerve (and gland). Physical attitude and mental attitude come together in muscle tone.

It is also clear to athletes, if not to physiologists, that gamma system activity stimulates the hypothalamus. Not only does an elevated mood increase gamma system activity, but gamma system activity—exercise, physical movement, deliberate firing of the muscle spindles—elevates mood. Stretching fires the muscle spindles. Stretching, I am tempted to say, will make you happy. Happier, anyway. Stretch away your blues.

I'm sure of this (experientially); the physiologists aren't. It is a speculative leap too large for the cautions of science. To explain exercise's effect on mood, scientists have recently been more interested in endorphins—as in "runner's high." (They're not finding quite as large a phenomenon as they expected.) It seems unlikely, however, that this connection between hypothalamus and gamma system, no matter how vague, could be a one-way street.

Physiology regularly describes discrete link-ups as if they exist so simply, but of course they never do. On any spinal cord motor nerve there are something like six thousand connections. Every nerve cell is enmeshed in an unimaginable web of filtering, modulation, feedback. One-way circuits, like all-or-none responses, exist only in laboratory dissections. Surely, stretching of the muscle spindles excites the hypothalamus and elevates the mood. As surely as movement makes you feel better. Everybody knows that, except scientists.

MOVEMENTS BRILLIANT AND NOT SO BRILLIANT

The muscle spindle helps you make that graceful figure-8 wave of the hand, but not without the aid of the other proprioceptors. Proprioception, too, is all one piece. It is the complex means by which we take a bombardment of information and turn it into all that is purposeful and accurate—and therefore beautiful—in the way we use our bodies.

It can get out of whack. If you've been in a cast, bedridden, or otherwise movement-deprived, you know how that feels. When you start moving again, you don't quite know where anything *is*, or how hard, how far, even in which direction to make any move. Lack of movement is a progressive disease, as the elderly often discover; movement not only loses its pleasure but becomes anxious-making. That's how couch potatoes are born: their proprioceptors go to sleep. People who begin to exercise after a long layoff perceive their bodies as broader and heavier than they actually are, and movement as more effortful. Even if you're active, a change in exercise routine—from running to rowing, from endurance training to strength training—can change your self-perception, making you feel suddenly larger or smaller, lighter or heavier, more upright than usual. The change—usually a delightful one—happens because you start firing proprioceptors in unusual ways; it goes away when you habituate the proprioceptors to their new tasks. Getting your sea legs (*not* necessarily a pleasant change) and getting over them requires just such a proprioceptive adjustment.

Proprioception gets disordered from overuse and injury, too, and when it does it can cause endless muscle-tendon problems. Direct injury to proprioceptive nerve endings, or injury to surrounding tissue that changes the pressure or tension on the nerve endings, will send faulty information to the central nervous system, which then can't maintain the muscle in an appropriate state. The result can be a muscle that is *hypertonic*—tight, as athletes say—or *hypotonic*: simply weak, slow to react, inaccurate in its response. (*Reactive,* in chiropractic parlance.) A tight agonist muscle will often have a weakened antagonist; when one muscle isn't functioning properly, it stresses its connective tissue, the surrounding musculature that shares its load, and any involved joints—the rest of the one-piece body. Chronic muscular imbalance—from overdevelopment, overuse, even bad posture—can train your proprioceptors to send faulty information, increasing the imbalance. This, too, is a looped system.

Hard-used (and unstretched) muscles sometimes develop lumpy nodules of pain, ropy strips of fibrous material within the belly of the muscle, areas of increased density in the fascia, trigger points that refer pain elsewhere in the body. They are the athlete's legacy, and generally don't warrant serious concern from conventional medical science. They are usually associated in some way with proprioception gone awry. Stretching helps prevent some of these soft-tissue aberrations but isn't much more successful than anything else in getting rid of them. There are other ways of attacking them, discussed in chapter 8. These various treatment "modalities" are complex and difficult, and while some give good results—in some cases—they are quite often effective for a disappointingly short time, if at all.

Better to keep your proprioceptors healthy in the first place than to try to bring them back from dysfunction. Keeping them healthy and acute will make you a better athlete—or, if you're not athletic, simply more at ease in the physical world. You keep them fit as you do any other organ, with appropriate use. Appropriate use for these particular physical systems means taking them through their cycles of stretching and contraction. Conventional exercise starts the job but doesn't finish it. To stay supple, you have to supply additional stretching.

Listening to a violin concerto and thinking of these things, I am swept with speculative wonder at the proprioceptive pleasure of making such music happen. I am no musician, but I sing in the shower, and dance, now and then, across the kitchen floor. I find even these unskilled ventures into music pleasurable enough. They are proprioceptive thrills. It isn't your ears that give you pleasure when you sing, it's your throat, the muscles themselves, working smoothly and accurately to produce the sound you intend, sending messages of pleasure to your brain. Proprioception is the sense that allows you to hit the note you want.

I try to imagine being able to play the violin well. To use my fingers and hands and arms to make those sounds, to hit those notes with such firm accuracy and timing, to create such soaring joy. Imagine that pleasure. Yes, it takes understanding and intellect and all kinds of other mental and emotional input, but in the end, when it comes to making the music come out of the fiddle, it's proprioception, all proprioception, that does the job. The intelligence of the muscle. You know, that brute, stupid stuff.

PART III

THE LOSS OF

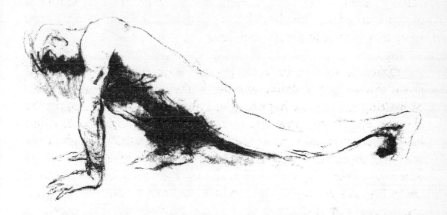

SUPPLENESS

EIGHT

BEYOND
STRETCHING

Loss of suppleness is loss of *homeostasis* of muscle and connective tissue. In medical terms, homeostasis is a state of equilibrium of the internal supplies of body fluids. Swelling, for instance, is a fluid imbalance. Spasms and knots in the tissue may result more from electrical than fluid imbalance: a disequilibrium of signaling. There are plenty of ways, wet and dry, for muscle and connective tissue to get out of sorts, and making them supple and strong again can be trickier than you expect. Sometimes just giving them time to heal isn't enough. Stretching helps, but it, too, can't fix everything.

When soft tissue gives serious trouble, orthodox medical treatment is indicated: remedy is most sensibly sought from orthopedia (or rheumatology, neurology, or some other medical specialty). But consider the possible range of soft tissue malfunction and discomfort: at one end the ordinary aches and pains of an active daily life, which stretching helps; at the other end, levels of injury or disease—fractures, severe sprains, tissue ruptures—that demand the attention of conventional medicine. In between are the minor tears and "pulls," low-grade variations on tendinitis, knots, spasms and other signs of outraged nerve endings, "cricks," "catches," and other inexplicable stiff places. Conventional medicine isn't very good at dealing with such annoyances. Over the centuries, we have developed a range of less intrusive and less orthodox therapies to challenge the range of musculoskeletal miseries. Some of them are efficacious, some are cuckoo. They're almost always ingenious, internally consistent—sometimes to the very edge of dementia—and more or less entertaining, which may help explain their enthusiastic followings.

Yoga is queen of them all, of course. Hatha yoga is a thousand-year-old discipline based on stretching and breathing. It is the physical practice associated with a classic form of Hindu philosophy. The yoga belief system is a structure of forbidding intricacy, but out of it has been carved a simplified program of postures and breathing exercises, performed to precise standards and rules. For all of these positions and exercises there are physiological rationales that make reasonable sense in Western terms. (The Eastern rationales are a little harder to penetrate.) Some instructors speak of hatha yoga as a science, but that characterization doesn't fit the Western definition of science very well.

Hatha yoga is a remarkably thorough internal self-exploration, aimed at cleansing the body of impurities and toning all its soft tissues; its adepts say it stimulates organs, glands, and nervous system as well. (The latter are also soft tissue, but beyond the scope of this book.) Some of the positions are quite rigorous, but there's an orderly progression toward them, to train the newcomer up to the required flexibility and strength. According to the yoga industry, instruction is very important; a lot of people nevertheless learn just enough to serve their individual needs, then go quietly off to practice regularly on their own.

Yoga is more than a physical discipline, it's a path, a way of life, its true purpose the search for enlightenment: perfection. My ambition isn't up to it. (My body sometimes wishes it were.) I confess, however, that I think of the approach to stretching in this book as a kind of American yoga, an attempt to seek out the purely pragmatic and concrete—and musculoskeletal—from the Indian discipline. A lot of hatha yoga is already in general use in physical therapy but isn't called by that name, in order not to scare people off. Properly performed, it can be a powerful aid to musculoskeletal health.

So can T'ai Chi. T'ai Chi Ch'uan has been characterized as moving yoga, which I find a seductive notion. It is a ritualized series of relaxed and flowing movements, timed to slow, deep breathing: a meditative dance. The legend of its origin is irresistible. It is said that aeons ago a Taoist hermit invented the movements as a way of getting the kinks out after a long day of sitting meditation in the cave. He wanted to restore his circulation and stretch out his soft tissues without interrupting his meditative concentration. I can't imagine a better approach to soft-tissue management. The movements are intended to represent natural phenomena: birds, animals, streams, clouds, and wind. They are lovely to watch, and strange.

Yoga and T'ai Chi are not so much therapies as practices, or, as their devotees might prefer, pathways. They are disciplines that, for all their poetic mystery, use the principles of exercise physiology for purposes of maintenance or improvement, and are self-applied. They are, in short, forms of athletic training, although their efforts and their ends are considerably subtler than we generally associate with athletic endeavor. Most other physical schemes are more remedial or corrective in concept. They range from the weird and loony to the utterly pleasurable: from aromatherapy, for example, to massage.

One of them is concerned specifically with stretching. Proprioceptive Neuromuscular Facilitation (PNF), a technique for improving flexibility and range of motion, is as close as we've come to a scientific approach to stretching; there is a body of research to support it, and it is widely used in clinical applications. Developed by Herman Kabat at the Kabat-Kaiser Institute in Vallejo, California, PNF has a complex physiological rationale, but in essence says that a muscle-tendon unit can be stretched farther if the stretch is interrupted for a brief isometric contraction, then stretched again. (An isometric contraction is one in which the muscle doesn't change in length, as when you pull against an immovable resistance.) The isometric contraction seems to reset the muscle spindles to accommodate the new, stretched-out length of the muscle. It is also thought to help inhibit the stretch reflex, facilitating greater relaxation.

The clinical version of the technique requires a stretching assistant. In the preferred therapeutic hamstring stretch, for instance, the patient lies supine and the therapist lifts the relaxed leg to stretch it. That's how therapists and physicians judge the tightness of hamstrings: by how high one leg can be raised before the other leg begins to be pulled up off the table. If the hamstring is tight and more range of motion is wanted, PNF techniques are applied. The therapist raises the passive leg to stretch the hamstring, then lowers it slightly to remove tension, and supports it there. The patient contracts the hamstring hard against this restraint. Then the hamstring is relaxed, and the therapist stretches it again. With repetition, the range of motion will increase.

This, if there is such a beast, is the scientific way to stretch. The implications for the casual stretcher, for those of us who simply want to stay supple, are unclear. If you know that a muscle-tendon group is tighter than it should be, figuring out a way to apply this technique to it makes sense. But I've known about PNF for years, I really believe in stretching, I've got some recognizable tight spots, but I almost never find myself applying PNF techniques. I'm not sure why.

As I write this, I give it a test. It's time for a break anyway: every hour or so I try to move away from my desk for a few minutes. When I do, the shoulder stretch in illustration 23 (p. 59) is a great relief for tired typing muscles. I try modifying it to make use of PNF principles. I stand in a doorway and do the stretch for a few seconds; relax; then grab the doorway behind me and contract the muscles of my breast for a moment or two, pressing outward on the doorjamb. I then relax and stretch again. Can't tell that much difference. Actually, now that I think about it, I alternately contract and relax those muscles when I'm doing this stretch anyway; it's a way of turning it from a position into a move, of working through its possibilities.

I'm not sure that PNF has much implication for the casual stretcher. It is used to good effect for rehabilitating injuries and for developing an unusual range of motion for special applications, such as dance or competitive athletics. I'm not sure an unusual range of motion is always a good idea. Most of the time the limitations to that range are in the joint capsule, and I'm not sure it's smart to try to increase it. Anyway, most of the stretching we do is (or ought to be) in relief of tension, not in pursuit of more range of motion. PNF is an extremely specific attack. Unless you are addressing a specific problem, you're better off with the one-piece-body approach.

Besides, if your stretches are moves instead of positions, if you roll around the joint as recommended in chapter 4, then you're applying a little PNF all the time anyway. To stretch one place is to contract someplace else—more or less isometrically—or you wouldn't be generating any tension. When your stretches are moves, you play the muscle back and forth between contraction and relaxation, in slow, gradual transitions from one state to the other. An isometric contraction is a hard-edged concept, but hardly the way we use our muscles in real life (unless what we set out to do specifically is an isometric contraction). Real-life use is a lot more complex and nonspecific than terms like isometric contraction describe; everyday stretching is a lot more complex and nonspecific—and therefore more complete—than sharply focused PNF. PNF is good therapy, but it's for specific deficits.

Massage, on the other hand, remains stubbornly impervious to scientific investigation, which doesn't keep it from being a perfectly wonderful tool for maintaining soft tissue health and suppleness. The problem with massage is that it uses the hands, and that means you've got soft tissue working on soft tissue. How are you going to hang any markers on that? Massage is too mushy for its numbers to be taken by scientists.

Conventional medicine traditionally ranks massage somewhere between astrology and voodoo. In athletics, American authorities have long regarded it as something of a European affectation. The highest levels of athletic management, however, have recently begun to come around. Particularly in individual sports such as track, swimming, and cycling, elite athletes are beginning to seek ways to travel and train with a personal masseur. The modern team-sport trainer's first choice for his bruised and battered charges is the whirlpool bath, but massage—much more thorough than the old "rub-down"—is becoming recognized as a worthwhile adjunct. Both whirlpool and massage gently manipulate the tissues to stimulate circulation, and therefore speed waste removal and repair. Serious athletes nowadays manage their bodies with a four-pronged attack: ice, whirlpool, massage, and stretching. Unfortunately, most of us non-elites can't afford or arrange regular treatment with whirlpool and massage. It's our loss. (I never pass up a chance at either one.)

Enthusiasts of massage speak of fabulous transactions taking place within the tissues as they work. Here is Rich Phaigh, for instance, masseur for the elite Athletics West track club (in *Athletic Massage,* Simon & Schuster, 1984):

> Massage loosens muscle fibers, separating them from one another so they can act freely, with more flexibility. It also helps lengthen muscles shortened by the frequent and hard contractions of athletics. It eliminates fatigue, promotes relaxation, relieves swelling, reduces muscle tension and helps prevent soreness. It can even speed recovery from injury. . . . Repeated deep massage aligns the cells of the scar tissue with the surrounding area. It gets rid of the rough edges of scar tissue by weaving the torn fibers back together. This eliminates the pain-causing irritation process that takes place when scar tissue comes into contact with healthy tissue. . . . Massage will also break adhesions formed between the scar and other muscles and will create fluid circulation inside the scar tissue to keep it soft.

He's speaking of athletic massage; there are about as many different forms and styles of massage as there are pairs of hands in the world, and I haven't got a bad word to say about any of them. You bang yourself somewhere, you rub the spot, right? And it feels a little better? That's massage: the principle starts there and goes right on up to schools and institutes and disciplines as complex as yoga, with elaborate (and sometimes unintentionally amusing) bodies of theory. Such codification is, in one sense, doomed: no two pairs of hands work exactly the same way, and no two upper backs or calves or hamstrings want exactly the same treatment, or accept it in the same way. And there, I groan to say it, is the rub: nothing can be quantified. The efficacy of the treatment depends on the skill of the practitioner. The hands are everything.

I'm not sure good hands can be taught. The term is used more often for the glue-fingered athlete, but anyone who gets his back rubbed knows that it applies as well to massage. For either purpose you need a high level of sensitivity to contour, texture, and density, a sure judgment about the application of force. Good hands are able to read fine distinctions and come up with just the right response to them. This is *stereognosis*—"shape knowledge," tactile recognition—and much more than merely a good sense of touch. It is another form of proprioception, that most athletic of capacities—whether it's used to haul in a hard-thrown wet football or to get at the knots in your back.

Getting at the knots is not the problem, unfortunately; getting rid of them is. Good hands have no trouble sniffing them out, and making wonderful things happen to them. The knots may even go away for a while. But if you resume the activity that put them there in the first place, they're likely to come back. That's one reason people keep inventing all these new techniques. They keep trying to come up with a cure for knots, spasms, tightnesses, and other products of overuse and low-grade injury. To do so would be to cure fatigue, to cure wear and tear; it isn't going to happen. (Living is a process, not a state.) If you try these treatments expecting a cure, you will be disappointed. If what you want is relief, almost all of these schemes more or less work, and sometimes wonderfully well. Ignore the claims, enjoy the product: applied kinesiology, osteopathy, chiropractic, manipulative therapy, deep-tissue massage, myotherapy, psychomuscular release therapy, shiatsu, rolfing, take your pick.

There is an enormous distance between massage and chiropractic, and it is patently unfair of me to lump all those treatments together that way. (And that's a very incomplete list.) Some are surely better than others, and the only real link between them may be that they involve human touch. Equating them so glibly is going to enrage a lot of their true believers. True believers tend to be a little testy anyway.

I've had considerable relief from chiropractic. It is my good fortune to have a friend named Keith McCormick who is a chiropractic physician and an athlete. He has a clearer sense of how the body works in vigorous activity than any A.M.A. doctor I've talked to, and he's been of immeasurable help to me with this book. Chiropractic is by far the most successful of the names in the list above, designating itself the largest drugless healing profession in the world. Conventional medicine has in the past dismissed chiropractic as quackery, although there is now growing cooperation between the two professions. (Conventional medicine also is in the business of seeking cures, with perhaps more success, and perhaps more catastrophic failures.)

Chiropractic is a complete body of medicine, far too comprehensive for a quick summary here. I wouldn't attempt to do so anyway; when I read its literature, I'm not sure I always follow. Chiropractic has an extensive theoretical foundation, but when it attempts to run science under that theory, it sometimes finds that it lives in a very difficult neighborhood in which to *do* science. A great deal of chiropractic's success (like surgery's) surely derives from good hands: proprioception, which is hard enough to measure, working with (or against) human feelings, which science can't even think about measuring. This is frustrating to chiropractic: it can provide relief but has trouble proving why that relief results from its ministrations.

I've been rolfed. (I've experienced some of the other drugless therapies, too, but not with particularly interesting results.) Rolfing is a technique of deep tissue massage, based on the assumption that the various traumas of our lifetimes are necessarily registered in our fascia. In response to injury, the fascia tightens, shortens, adheres to itself and to the muscles it covers. The processes of healing glue us together, but not always in the right places; the resulting distortion, plus the continuous effects of gravity, lead to misalignment and dysfunction, at least according to rolfing theory. Rolfing aims at ungluing us: at freeing up the fascia, lengthening shortened muscles, and generally putting the body right with gravity again. There are other, similar approaches to realigning and balancing the body structure by connective tissue manipulation, ringing more or less complex variations on the basic technique. Rolfing is the best known.

What rolfing is most famous for is being painful. (It was so satirized in the movie *Semi-Tough*.) I didn't find it so, but that may say more about faulty pain receptors than about rolfing. In any given session there would be a moment or two—perhaps fifteen or twenty seconds at a time—that I found distinctly unpleasant and wished were over with. But the rest of the hour was spent in the fiercest and most delicious massage I've ever experienced. I loved it so much that less than a year after completing the basic ten sessions, I went back for more.

I've read several anecdotal case histories of rolfing experiences, and my own is no different. The changes were most dramatic when they removed some anomaly that I'd accommodated unconsciously, that I didn't know I had. After one early session, I felt as if large rubber mounds had been shaved off the bottoms of my feet, their contact with the ground somehow much flatter and more secure. My hip sockets seemed to have been moved outward a couple of inches, giving me a wider stance. I felt more solidly grounded, more securely held to earth by gravity, yet lighter on my feet. I assume these changes in body image are caused by changes in proprioception: rolfing must free up the connective tissue around the proprioceptors, allowing them to fire in subtle new ways, ways forgotten in the gradual accretion of injury and scar tissue.

A lot of the changes were subjective, and therefore suspect, but I also gained, or regained, over an inch in height, and I've never considered height a subjective measurement. That is, rolfing did change things, which is something I cannot say about most of the other physical therapies (and a distressingly large part of the conventional medicine) I've experienced. It left me long and loose and full of juice. It did not get the knots out of my shoulders and back. I don't know how long its effects last, or whether it is a cure for anything. I went back for more sessions simply because I loved the way it felt.

The technique is hard to describe. There's a lot of deep digging, lifting, separating of the flesh, with thumbs and knuckles. A primary technique involves sliding an elbow slowly, with considerable pressure, down the length of the muscle. Rolfing, too, is a kind of stretching: microstretching, so to speak, at the level of muscle and connective tissue fibers, and at angles and in directions that ordinary stretching—restricted to the lines of force through which the muscle-tendon units work—can't achieve. If rolfing is a kind of stretching, so is Rich Phaigh's athletic massage, of course, and most of the other touching therapies we've invented to ease aching flesh. Unfortunately, these therapies tend to break into warring camps, factionalism, cults of personality. The rancor is too bad: connective tissue seems to be helped by the treatments, never mind the ideology. Soft tissue just seems to want to be *worked:* worked on, as well as worked with.

Quackery, sniffs the M.D.; logic (and sensitivity), claims the practitioner. Good hands, says I. It's also too bad that working with your hands on someone is slow, effortful, and unprofitable. Most conventional therapists don't want to use their hands, they want to use machines, which not only take less time and sweat but also somehow make the bill more palatable. As the costs of conventional medicine soar, hand work is left more and more to the unconventional. Sometimes it's hard to tell the merely unorthodox from the wackos. Too many of them talk too good a game.

There have been people healing—or helping, anyway—with their hands since we got up off all fours and found our hands available for touching one another. The ones who've been the best at this kindness have always tried to pass their special talents on. Too often this seems to require draping mystery over the subject. Sometimes the mystery has been technical, sometimes theosophical. All the mystery in the world doesn't add or subtract a whit from good hands, though, or the amount of relief to be had therefrom.

The problem comes when people make a cult out of the source of that relief. People try to make a cult out of stretching, too. That's just as silly.

SHRINKAGE

Man is as old as his connective tissues.
—Alexander A. Bogomoletz, Ukrainian physician
and scientist, 1881–1946

No point in kidding about it: age is a large personal concern of mine. I'm in my mid-fifties, I compete in masters athletics, I receive daily reminders of shrinking physical capacities. Not that my concern is unique, or even a product of my particular antiquity: if you're past the age of consent—particularly if you are athletic—you already have a problem with aging. While it is true that peak performances can occur later in some disciplines than in others, the physiological underpinnings of those performances cannot indefinitely be improved. At some undetermined point—usually in the third decade of life—one's physical promise begins to shrink. This shrinkage is not just an athletic problem: what's sauce for the athlete is sauce for the merely active. It gets us all: nobody is immune. And sure enough, the legs really do go first.

Aging is a very real but mysterious process. A committee of the AMA spent ten years considering the problem of human aging, and concluded that it could find no physical or mental condition that could be directly attributed to the passage of time.

That is, we know fairly well what aging does to us, but we don't really know what it is about aging that does it. There seems to be some kind of genetic clock in living creatures. Human cell cultures will divide about fifty times before they die off. Freeze the cultures after twenty divisions, and you stop the process in its tracks; thaw them again and they will divide about thirty more times, and die. Something seems to keep count.

One theory blames accumulated genetic damage, from radiation or other sources, which is assumed to interfere with accurate replication and repair. The thymus gland generally shrinks with age, and when it does, the immune system also loses effectiveness, decreasing our resistance to disease. The connection is unclear. There are nutritional and environmental theories of aging. Lab rats live longer if they eat less; fish live longer in cold water; frogs that mature in one season at sea level can take two or three seasons to mature at alpine altitudes. Growing seasons are keyed not only to time but to heat and light. Nobody says that life isn't a temporary condition, but nobody knows why that should be so.

There are plenty of antiaging theories, too—"schemes" might be a better word—and exercise leads the pack. If you look at aging as a disease, it is one of *hypokinesis:* too little movement. Loss of function is the only unpleasant part of aging; everything else is fine, even enjoyable. Function is maintained by use. Whatever aging is and whatever may cause it, its deleterious effects are best resisted actively. Use it or lose it: Hippocrates propounded this theory over two thousand years ago, and gerontologists have found no reason to abandon it.

If you enjoy physical activity, it's a terrific theory. The fitness craze is largely based on it (or that part of the fitness craze that isn't based on weight control, i.e., appearance, or sex). I took a heavy position in it myself about ten years ago, undertaking a fairly extensive personal investigation of its application (*Staying With It,* Viking, 1984). There's a body of scientific literature indicating that losses in physiological capacity associated with aging can be slowed, halted, or even reversed by sufficient exercise. This literature comes largely out of exercise physiology, a discipline whose range of measurements is limited and, undoubtedly, biased. But for clinical treatment of the deleterious effects of aging, the hypokinetic approach is just about the only game in town.

In *Staying With It* I summarized the expected physiological progression of hypokinesis: loss of overall height, sitting height, shoulder width, and chest depth (but for some reason age makes the nose, ears, and hat size grow larger); loss of muscle mass, rise in body fat; loss of bone strength, lung function, and joint elasticity. Loss of cardiac output. General wastage of metabolically active tissue. (Shortening muscles cause skeletal changes, impinge on blood flow, and decrease oxygen supplies not only to the muscles but to the brain.) Motor nerve responsiveness slows, decreasing our coordination, stability of movement, balance. We get clumsy, and when we injure ourselves, we heal more slowly. But more than anything else, what aging seems to do is dry us up. In the lens of the eye, in the disks that stabilize the spine, in the joints, even in the mouth and the digestive tract, loss of fluid is the characteristic change associated with age. Fluid is our best lubricant; without it we quickly stiffen.

Activity, according to the exercise physiologists, will resist, if not reverse, these changes. But activity is use, and connective tissue is unfortunately vulnerable to both under- and overuse. With connective tissue, aging doubles the ante, setting a particularly clever trap. Underuse lowers the level at which the structural fatigue of overuse sets in. Overuse isn't the opposite of aging, it's another kind of aging, to which underuse makes you more vulnerable. Inactivity narrows the range of use within which connective tissue can continue to function in healthy fashion.

The older you get, the more gently (but faithfully) you must push against the limits to that range. Stretching is the most controllable tool you have for working the limits back, restoring the range. The older you get, the more you need to stretch. The older you get, the better stretching feels. I'm old enough to guarantee this.

ANOTHER TREATISE ON COLLAGEN

*A Treatise on Collagen** is the title of a multivolume medical text devoted entirely to that fundamental building block. There's good reason for such extensive treatment: as the *Treatise* points out, "Collagen in the form of insoluble fibers or fibrous aggregates represents the major proteinaceous constituent of most vertebrates and many invertebrates." While all those volumes do present perhaps more about collagen than you might ever want to know, they also give a thorough picture of what happens to connective tissue as it ages.

Collagen is currently at risk of becoming a buzz-word. Cosmetics manufacturers and other dream purveyors are now advertising its inclusion in their products. Smearing fibers of protein on your skin is somehow supposed to make your wrinkles go away. (Why do I keep remembering that famous ad line, "Bolivian tin miners don't get acne"?) It's not an unlikely association, even to cosmetologists: skin *is* mostly collagen. Unfortunately, an effective means of resisting or reversing skin's obvious aging processes has proved elusive. No matter what you put on it, skin tone tells as much about someone's age, at first glance, as anything else: more, for example, than whitening hair or a balding head, both of which can be premature. Your hide, out there in the weather and the rays, is what gives your age away. Our vanity may stuff the pockets of the skin-care industry, but our money hasn't bought a breakthrough yet. If it had, we wouldn't still be estimating age by the dermal evidence.

When skin ages, what happens to it is that it *tans,* pure and simple—not in color but in the literal sense of turning into leather. All those wrinkles, splotches, changes in thickness, sags and pouches, are products of its leatherization. Science's investigations of skin

*Bernard S. Gould, ed., Academic Press, London & New York, 1968.

and its aging processes actually began with trade information from the tanning industry. Tanning is the process that turns flesh into leather: it turns moist living material—soft and flexible but subject to decay if its nutrient supply is interrupted—into a drier, stronger, more tightly woven stuff. The new material is more susceptible to structural fatigue. I am describing my own face and, to one degree or another, yours. I could also be describing aging tendons.

Aging's effect on external connective tissue may be more dramatic, but similar processes are going on inside. (Alcohol, by the way, contains many chemicals used in tanning; cirrhosis is a kind of tanning of the liver. Tobacco smoke has been used to tan tendon material in labs; emphysema is tanning of the lungs.) Earlier, I likened connective tissue to wet fiberglass, with collagen and elastin as the fibers and the mucopolysaccharide ground substance as the uncongealed glass—a kind of lubricant to allow the microfibrils to work freely and flexibly. When connective tissue ages, the glass begins to harden. The "gel-to-fiber ratio" changes, the proportion of ground substance diminishing while collagen and elastin increase. The ground substance begins to dry out, to lose its lubricity, while the fibers become thicker, stronger, and less elastic.

This thickening of fibers, the single most characteristic physical change from aging, is caused by *cross-linking*. The fibers are twisted strands of protein molecules, bundled together by hydrogen bonds known as cross-links. New, healthy collagen doesn't have many links: the fibers are free to work independently. With aging, cross-linkage increases, forming additional hydrogen bonds both within and between the molecules in the collagen fibers. The fibers become more organized and less soluble. They are gradually glued together into clumps of larger diameter. The thicker fibers lose a certain amount of flexibility and begin to generate greater friction as they work. They gain great strength but they lose suppleness. They become relatively inert and less adaptable to change, less accessible to the remodeling and resorption by which the body normally repairs itself.

Tanning is, essentially, cross-linking. Some scientists regard cross-linkage and aging as almost synonymous terms. The *Treatise* presents the hypothesis that aging is "no more than an unfortunate biological accident brought about by the tanning of tissue proteins, including collagen, by metabolic products and other ingested substances potentially capable of inducing cross-linkage." Collagen's primary role in aging goes like this:

> During maturation there are readily demonstrable changes in the collagen of connective tissue. The aggregation and cross-linkage of collagen increases throughout the life-span.
>
> This aggregation and cross-linkage of collagen eventually reaches a point where it is incompatible with normal physiological function. This process either initiates or establishes the rate of aging. Specifically, there is interference with the diffusion of nutrients, oxygen, and waste products between cells, leading to death and aging.
>
> The principal cause of death in the human species is cardiovascular disease. The over-maturation of collagen predisposes the cardiovascular system to pathological deterioration.
>
> If the rate of collagen cross-linkage could be modified the human life-span could be extended.*

All you can really do about cross-linkage, unfortunately, is fight it. The genius of the jogging revolution, of Dr. Kenneth Cooper's whole aerobic invention, is that it specifically fights this pathological deterioration of the cardiovascular system. Systematically raising the heart and respiratory rates maintains or increases their capacity even in the face of aging. It does so not only by developing or maintaining their musculature but also by resisting the overmaturation of their collagen: by giving their connective tissue a good stretch. Aerobic exercise helps maintain the suppleness of the cardiovascular system.

Cardiovascular deterioration isn't the only problem. Elsewhere,

*Gould, vol. 2, Biology of Collagen, Part B.

discussing healing and tissue repair, the *Treatise* makes a more startling case that there are a variety of age-dependent degenerative diseases that at the most basic level involve collagenous tissue: "There are no grounds, at present, for doubting that hepatic cirrhosis, nephrosclerosis, arteriosclerosis, arthritis and many other so-called 'degeneratory' and 'auto-immune' diseases have, as a major (if not as *the* major) component, the formation of new collagen, often ultimately almost indistinguishable histologically from cutaneous scars."*

You might say we live our normal lives in a state of low-grade fibrosis, which aging gradually exacerbates. Maturation tries to "heal" our hard-used connective tissue into a stronger, denser material. We stiffen and shrink—and, eventually, die. The longer we manage to hang on to our suppleness, the longer we live, the better we function.

The rate at which cross-linkage occurs can perhaps be slowed. There are chemical as well as mechanical approaches. It is probably worth the effort to control whatever environmental factors you can. You should remember that the "suntan" doesn't refer to the color: your skin will stay younger if you don't deliberately tan it with exposure to the sun. If there is an effective elixir of youth, cosmetically speaking, it isn't ground-up collagen in grease, it's octyl dimethyl PABA, the sun-blocking ingredient in contemporary sun lotions.

There is also, I'm sure, a nutritional approach to the delay of cross-linking, although whether it is more effective than smearing protein fibers on your face may be open to question. There is a nutritional approach to almost everything these days, although most of them require a certain willing suspension of disbelief. You can find anything you want in nutrition: it has become the new astrology.

The only other alternative I know of for purposes of fighting cross-linkage is the mechanical one, which, in one form or another, involves stretching. The kind of stretching presented in the

*Gould, vol. 2.

previous chapters admittedly addresses only the major musculo-skeletal aspects of the inexorably aging system. But that's the very part that lets you continue to lead an active life.

AGING ATHLETES

I became a competitive athlete in my late forties and wrote about the physiological results in *Staying With It*. Since that book was published, I've revised my understanding of age and aging. I'm still applying the principles, but I now expect, and get, rather different results.

One powerful stimulus to that project was the aforementioned body of research saying that hard training can maintain, if not improve, the standard measurements of exercise physiology, and can do so more or less indefinitely. Studies of the general population show a decline in maximum oxygen uptake, for instance, of about one percent per year; athletes who have continued to train intensely enough, however, have maintained or even improved their maximum oxygen uptake over decades.

In training to resist aging, intensity seems to be more important than volume, which leads to a certain amount of self-selection in such longitudinal studies. Athletes who are able to maintain the intensity of their efforts over decades are those who are able to avoid injuries from either overuse or trauma. They are athletes who are blessed with, or somehow develop, exceptionally good connective tissue, among other things. In my case, which is not in any way rare, I loved the intensity but my connective tissue didn't. To train intensely enough to attain peak performances was to break down. I have had to learn the limits of my connective tissue, which turn out to be lower than the limits to performance that I want to accept. This particular price of aging—a disappointment, not a tragedy—is not the sort of thing that exercise physiology measures. Aging turns out to be real, all right, even when you maintain your physiological measurements.

Stretching does not erase this disappointment, but I've found that it materially lessens it, now that I know what I'm doing. This has taken a while. When I began stretching I followed the standard manuals, with considerable frustration; none of them told me enough to understand what I was doing. As those manuals presented stretching, it helped, but not enough. When training intensity began to outrun my connective tissue's resilience, I realized that stretching wasn't doing as much for me as it should. That's when I began figuring out what stretching ought to be, what I ought to be doing. That's when I began stretching for pleasure, not for a position in a stretching book. Rehabilitation is a wonderful teaching device.*

Now, I use stretching as a first-line specific, against the first hint of musculoskeletal disequilibrium—just as soon as I get finished using it for pleasure. I recently returned from a winter vacation that involved several kinds of unaccustomed vigorous activity. It was a busy time and I didn't always get my stretching in. If I stretched out the unaccustomed but hard-used soft tissues, I didn't get sore; if I didn't stretch, I got sore, as regular as clockwork. I found myself amused at the predictability. I don't know why this surprised me: if I skip a couple of days of stretching during my regular, routine days, I get stiff and mildly sore. It makes me feel old.

It should be obvious by now that I think stretching is a miracle cure-all for mankind's ills and the likely eventual source of world peace. Bolivian tin miners don't get acne, either. I've tried to provide the physiological rationale for benefits to be derived from stretching, but to do so without making claims. I have nothing on which to base claims but my own experience,

---

*But a neglected one. I've had two fractures and assorted sprains requiring medical attention and have never been given the first word of advice about rehabilitating them. I know of an athlete who had arthroscopic surgery to his knee, and was not given exercises to regain its strength and mobility until he demanded them, weeks after the surgery. Nonorthopedic health professionals have told me worse horror stories. I've never known *anyone*—except an occasional elite athlete—who has been instructed by an M.D. to rehabilitate an injury. Nobody I know has even been advised by the medical profession to exercise.

and I wouldn't expect anyone to accept that as the basis for anything. You have to try these things for yourself. According to the standard formula for such internally consistent but outwardly nutty schemes, stretching should cure all. It doesn't. It's just a handy, comfortable, and totally pleasurable way to help in the management of soft tissue. The only claim I make is that stretching feels good. For some people. I'm particularly grateful that I happen to be one of them.

I'm talking about stretching as a form of gentle exercise to help maintain the suppleness of the musculoskeletal system. Macro-stretching, you might call it: external stretching. More conventional exercise, aerobic or otherwise, might be considered internal, or micro-stretching; clearly, it, too, involves a systematic resistance to cross-linking/tanning/aging of the soft tissues. That's a health benefit from exercise that hasn't had much attention, but it certainly seems a worthy line of thought. In any event, this is not a whimsical area of consideration. The *Treatise on Collagen* calls the general hardening of connective tissue, in all its various forms, the most important unresolved problem in pathology and medicine.

> *Hamlet:* How long will a man lie i' the earth ere he rot?
>
> *Gravedigger:* . . . he will last you some eight year or nine year: a tanner will last you nine year.
>
> —*Act V, Scene I*

TEN

PHYSICS—AND A LITTLE COACHING

Staying supple requires that you keep your connective tissue healthy. You do that by giving it an appropriate level of use. Appropriate use means, among other things, avoiding traumatic loading. You avoid traumatic loading by doing things the easy way. For people who enjoy physical effort, this may be the hardest lesson of all to learn. I find myself learning it again, in some small way, nearly every day of my life.

It's silly to have such trouble getting it through my head. The benefits accrue not just to the connective tissue but to the efforts themselves. Coaches tell us this in a thousand ways: relax, stop trying so hard, take a little off, stay within yourself, don't press, stay loose, take your time, get it right. More moves go bad because they're launched too early than because they're too late. As a canny old pro once told me, you have to have the confidence to take the time. The complexity of this athletic truth grows on me daily. And it sounds so simple.

The coaches are saying that the easy way is the best way: it's the way that everything *works* best (including your connective tissue). It's easiest because you've got the physical details right— accurate, aligned, well timed. When you do that, you protect the connective tissue from traumatic loading. You also end up getting more speed or force or whatever it was you wanted from the move in the first place. The move *really* works. Click: sweet spot.

Formal athletic instruction is sometimes referred to as physical education. *Physical* comes from *physics*. An athlete is in the business of making judgments about physical laws in real time. It helps to remember that: athletic tasks are problems in practical physics, involving acceleration, deceleration, momentum and mass, vectors of force, all those elements of mechanical law. (In your imagination, run a little footage of the hammer throw.) Hockey player Wayne Gretzky isn't as big or fast or strong as his opponents, but he's far better at his given task than anyone else in the sport. When asked how this can be, he points out that you can pass the puck faster than you can skate with it. "My game is all angles," he says. He's talking physics—and it's the physics of skate blade against ice as well as stick against puck.

Gretzky generates a lot of sportswriterly analysis. He has been tested scientifically and found to be physically ordinary, with no offscale attributes to explain his edge. Sportswriters usually explain him by reciting his statistics; pushed for a nonnumerical assessment, they leap from the physical to the metaphysical. Gretzky's uncanny skills have been credited, for example, to exceptional vision, not in acuity or peripheral range or other measurable optical aspect but in some mysterious additional quality—rink sense, for want of a better term. He plays, they say, as if he sees what's happening everywhere on the ice at once, among all the players, no matter where he's looking. He simply knows what's going on, selects his next move unerringly from the dizzying multitude of possibilities, seems always to be two or three plays ahead of everyone else.

These capacities make for terrific hockey but don't offer a very fruitful way to understand the sport. Describing them doesn't tell much about what athleticism really is, and it is pure athletic ability—the actual source of Wayne Gretzky's advantage—that is the basic currency of the sports world. This is a problem. In the meat markets of the pros, where there is much to lose from fuzzy judgments, they look for special skills first, stats second, and after that they always say they're looking for the best available athlete.

End of discussion: nobody ever says what that is. They speak of athleticism as one of those vague qualities like character or leadership. Or rink sense.

But the pros know exactly what they're looking for in that third category, even if they can't define it. The fans do too. We know a Gretzky when we see one. There is simply a quality of movement, a silken easiness, that arrests the eye. A lot of superstars don't quite have it, and a lot of athletes who have it in abundance have disappointing careers, but it's worth watching—it's almost impossible not to watch—wherever it occurs. The best available athlete is the one who has more of this quality of movement than his or her peers. It is movement in which the physics have been gotten right. It indicates an instinct, a natural flair, for the easy solution to the rapidfire problems in physics that constitute athletic activity. It is the single quality that translates from sport to sport, since all sports abide by the same physical laws.

Dennis Golden is a former diver, a Ph.D. in biomechanics, and the head of the technical committee of the organization that governs diving in the U.S. On my way to a Greg Louganis practice session, I asked him what to look for. "Just watch," Golden said. "You're going to see the most *efficient* athlete in the world today." I can't come up with a nominee to challenge that statement.

It struck me that Golden didn't say anything about beauty, although beauty and perfection are the words people usually use to describe Louganis's performances, and what he does is surely as beautiful as any athletic activity ever devised. This focus on efficiency is hardly a revolutionary idea: even Plato told us that the most beautiful motion will be that which accomplishes the greatest results with the least effort. Get efficient enough and the beauty part will take care of itself. What we respond to visually in athletics is the startling efficiency of the exactly appropriate move—whether it is by Louganis or Gretzky or Carl Lewis. The right move is, always, the loveliest moment in sports.

It's more thrilling to make that move than to watch it, of

course, which is why we play all these games. Nearly forty years ago I tried to be a diver myself, and did manage, however infrequently, to "rip" a dive now and then—to enter the water so vertically and well aligned that there was virtually no splash. I remember clearly what that was like. You prepare yourself for the shock of hitting the water, but it never arrives. You don't hit the water, you simply touch it and it closes around you, swallowing you without resistance. You penetrate so quickly and so hard that you risk smashing into the bottom of the pool. It is a glimpse, each time, of an effortless world in which all the alignments are right, the forces properly aimed, the leverage perfect. Your body instantly yearns to go back, do it again, spend more time in that effortless world. It's a haunting experience, but there's nothing mystical about it. It's just that for once you really did get the physics right.

As a journalist I've also covered motor racing, skiing, the high jump, the pole vault, gymnastics, swimming. The coaches and athletes all say the same thing, however the terminology differs. Success in these very different disciplines comes from getting the physics right. It is the common principle of athletic effort—and of the performing arts. The best performers—the Itzhak Perlmans and Mikhail Baryshnikovs as well as the Martina Navratilovas—are those who put the physics of the world to the best use.

Proprioception is the sense that helps you get the physics right; biomechanics is the study of the cost of getting the physics wrong. Its study is the physics of physiology. Much biomechanical research involves high-speed photography of athletic motions, usually from several angles simultaneously, with markers carefully placed on the joints, force plates attached to the limbs. If you surround the athletic motion with external sensors for distance, force, rate, and anything else you can figure out how to measure, you can record much of the same sort of information that the proprioceptors sense. If you can record it, you can turn it into math, and solve it. Biomechanics is the analytical tool that is expected to solve all questions of athletic technique. Until the next gross-motor genius comes along and figures out—*feels* out, proprioceptively—a better way.

Formal athletic technique, as taught by coaches and instructors, is the accumulated wisdom of the best observers of the sport, codified into the idealized version of the way the idealized human form would perform the task. Your personal technique—in swimming, skiing, tennis, or any other athletic activity—is your own best effort at matching the consensus view of the experts, modified by the specifics of your particular physical plant. It's your biomechanical solution for your particular kit of bone lengths, joint angles, muscular attachment points.

If your technique is bad, your athletic efforts will be inefficient—and your connective tissue will eventually get hurt. Good technique means operating from a firmly established center of gravity with solid purchase and traction, eliminating wasted motion, applying force smoothly and in straight lines, keeping motions compact (to reduce the chance of introducing extraneous angles), finishing off each move (to get your weight in the right place for the next), and so on. Bad technique means more effort is required for the same result: energy is wasted in wrong directions, joints pounded at bad angles, tendons and ligaments yanked and brutalized, unnecessary tensions transmitted throughout the one-piece body.

Bad equipment, or congenital bad alignment of muscles and joints, can cause your technique to be bad no matter how you try to correct it. Even if your technique and your equipment are as mechanically sound as you can make them, you still may suffer overuse injuries. You injure connective tissues when you apply tension too quickly, unexpectedly, at the wrong angle, when they are already loaded or stretched. The more you are off the mark in an athletic movement, the more you load the connective tissues. Even if you have the movement precisely right, if you continue with muscles stiffened by fatigue, you risk injury.

Mechanical solutions—tape, braces, orthotics—are external ways of helping you get the physics right. If you are injured, you *will* improve your technique, or you will abandon that part of it that caused the injury. Or you will suffer recurring injuries. To graduate from tape and braces—whether you are rehabilitating an injury or trying to avoid injury in the first place—you have to condition the required muscle-tendon units to be strong enough to handle the tensile forces without suffering overload, and to have enough stamina to maintain their suppleness throughout the task. The better your physics, however, the lighter the loading, the less the risk.

To stay supple, it behooves you to seek out good physics: to work to find the smoothest and easiest technique for any activity you undertake. Or, as I must keep repeating to the idiot who uses my body, you don't stay supple by going at things as if you are killing snakes.

No one is gifted with the ability always to get the physics right, but I think we are athletic to the degree that we choose to try. We are athletic to the degree that we understand the world in those terms: that it is a physical world, susceptible to our manipulation, and that the more accurate that manipulation, the easier—and more satisfying—the result. Most of a child's play is devoted to working out the physics of the world, the weights and measures. Even the littlest kids are also solving problems in time, rate, and distance, and how their growing bodies fit into those equations. A one-year-old learning to toddle is a practical physicist at work in the lab, trying to learn to operate the world a little better. You don't stop being an athlete until you quit trying to learn that.

The better you learn to operate the world—to take a little off, to relax and get it right—the better off your connective tissue will be. The more supple you will be.

The critic dismisses opera singers as "truckdrivers," "mere athletes." Curious attitude. Oh, they're athletes, all right. They perform muscular feats of great effort and fine control over extended periods of time—for which, of course, they train harder than many more-conventional athletes. They perform repertoire specifically composed to demonstrate the highest achievements of the human voice, and they do so to a critical standard about five times tougher than any applied in sports. Opera singers are fabulous athletes. There's nothing "mere" about them.

Calling them truckdrivers implies that they just deliver the notes, the sounds. And hold up some fancy costumes. I assume the carping critic wants artists rather than athletes: more sensitive souls who will somehow deliver more intellectual or emotional content in their performances, something beyond the merely physical. It's a peculiarly arrogant requirement, implying that the attempt to sing as well as humanly possible isn't noble enough.

If performers are athletes, perhaps the critic ought to check in with a coach. Any good coach could tell him that it's when you attempt to lay something extra on top of the pure performance of the task—extra force, speed, effort, intelligence, emotion—that things go bad. That's when ego starts getting in the way of the physics. Even a critic should be able to understand that the truest way, in the carpenter's sense of straight lines and sound alignments, is the truest way aesthetically, even philosophically. And seeking that kind of truth is what athletes do.

"Emotions have nothing to do with it," says Bob Dylan, in his enigmatic way. Emotion is not something you put in or take out. Get the task right (get it true) and the emotion takes care of itself. The great musicians learn, in the end, just to play the notes: to seek to demonstrate not the artist's skill but the music's content. Knowing that if the music is made clear, the passion and intelligence—of performer as well as of composer—will shine through. Truly.

Besides, playing it that way is easier on your connective tissue.

GLOSSARY

Achilles tendon—The tendon connecting calf muscle to heel bone.

Actin—Strands of protein that make up the thin filaments within the muscle fiber. When the muscle contracts, the thin and the thick (*myosin*) filaments slide alongside each other, interdigitating.

Aerobic—Oxygen-using. In current usage, exercise at a pace at which oxygen supply keeps up with oxygen use.

Afferent nerve—A nerve that carries signals—usually sensory information—toward the brain. Opposed to *efferent*.

Agonist—The muscle that is the prime power source for a particular move.

Antagonist—The muscle opposite the one in use. When you flex a joint, the flexors are agonists and the extenders are antagonists; when you extend a joint, the roles are switched.

Ballistic—Having to do with the behavior of missiles in flight. In exercise physiology, ballistic movements are those initiated by muscular contraction and completed by momentum, such as throwing and kicking. "Ballistic stretching" is stretching by jerking on the tissue.

Calisthenics—Ballistic stretching.

Cardiorespiratory—The system of heart and lungs that gets oxygen into and carbon dioxide out of the body.

Cardiovascular—The system of heart, arteries, and veins that circulates blood through the body.

Chiropractic—A system of healing based on the theory that disease results from failure of normal nerve function.

Collagen—Strands of protein that give connective tissue its tensile strength.

Concentric—In muscle contraction, when the muscle works by shortening.

Connective tissue—What ties you together into one flexible piece: tendon, ligament, fascia, skin, the covering material for organs, muscles, and bones.

Cross-linkage—The increase in hydrogen bonding between protein molecules in connective tissue fibers, usually from aging, which decreases the tissue's suppleness by increasing its density, stiffness, and susceptibility to injury.

Cross-training—Training in one athletic discipline in hopes of improving in another.

Eccentric—In muscle contraction, when the muscle works against a lengthening force, as when lowering a weight.

Efferent nerve—A nerve that carries signals from the central nervous system toward the extremities, signalling for action: a motor nerve. Opposed to *afferent*.

Elasticity—The capability of recovering shape after deformation. As used here, implying a certain springy storage of energy that speeds the rebound after deformation.

Elastin—Fibers of protein that give connective tissue its elasticity.

Extend—To straighten a joint; the opposite of flex.

Fascia—The fibrous membrane that covers, supports, and separates the muscles.

Fast-twitch muscle fiber—"White" muscle fiber, used primarily for quickness and strength, with limited endurance. See *Slow-twitch muscle fiber.*

Fatigue—Exhaustion of physiological resources.

Fibrosis—Abnormal formation of fibrous tissue. One response of muscle and connective tissue to the microtrauma of hard use.

Fitness—A level of physical health and conditioning suitable for the demands of one's chosen activities. (A marathoner isn't more "fit" than a sprinter, only more fit for distance running.)

Flex—To bend; the opposite of extend.

Flexibility—The ability to bend or stretch without damage; see *Suppleness* and *Elasticity.*

Gamma system—The neural loop connecting muscle spindle to central nervous system to muscle mass, with both afferent and efferent nerves.

Gastrocnemius—The superficial calf muscle, which overlies the soleus.

Golgi tendon organ—A proprioceptor that reads the amount of tension on the tendon.

Hamstring—The group of muscles and tendons at the back of the thigh, tying buttock to lower leg, responsible for extending the upper leg and flexing the lower leg.

Hypertonic—A dysfunctional muscle state, the muscle literally "tight": too much muscle tone, incapable of being fully relaxed.

Hypotonic—The opposite of hypertonic: flaccid, weak, unresponsive, inhibited from full contraction.

Isometric contraction—A muscle contraction that generates force against a constant length, as when you pull against an immovable object. An *isotonic contraction*, by contrast, generates a constant tension whatever the length of the muscle.

Joint capsule—The bag of connective tissue that encapsulates the joint and contains its lubricating (synovial) fluids.

Ligament—The connective tissue that attaches the bones to one another.

Microtrauma—Microscopic ruptures of muscle and connective tissue from hard use.

Motor nerve—A nerve that stimulates muscle fibers to contract.

Motor unit—One motor nerve and all the muscle fibers it serves. Thus, the unit of muscular reaction stimulated by a single nerve signal.

Muscle spindle—A proprioceptor that senses muscle length, change of length, and rate of change of length, and thereby maintains muscle tone, operates the stretch reflex, and governs style of movement.

Muscle tear—Rupture of muscle fibers and their enclosing connective tissue. Muscle tears occur most frequently at the attachment of muscle to tendon, less frequently within the muscle fiber. When muscle fiber does rupture, the point of separation is where the thin (actin) filaments attach to the Z line.

Musculoskeletal—The system of muscles, bones, tendons, and ligaments that permits active motion.

Myofibril—The smallest unit of muscle fiber, made up of strands of actin and myosin.

Myosin—Strands of protein that make up the thick filaments within the muscle fiber. When the muscle contracts, thick and thin (actin) filaments slide alongside each other, interdigitating.

Neuromuscular—The system of nerves and muscles that controls both voluntary and reflexive movement.

Overuse—Levels of use that exceed the organism's capacity to recover.

Pacinian corpuscle—A proprioceptor that senses movement and rate of change, located in the joint.

Progressive overload—A training technique based on the organism's capacity to respond to stress, over time, by increasing its capacity.

Proprioception—Self-sensing: the "continuous but unconscious sensory flow from the movable parts of our body (muscles, tendons, joints), by which their position and tone and motion is continually monitored and adjusted." (Oliver Sacks, *The Man Who Mistook His Wife for a Hat*.)

Proprioceptive neuromuscular facilitation—A therapeutic technique for increasing range of motion, using stretching exercises interspersed with brief, ultraspecific muscle contractions.

Psoas—The muscle group that connects spine to groin across the front of the pelvis.

Quadriceps—The group of four muscles at the front of the thigh, responsible for flexing the upper leg and extending the lower leg.

Range of motion—How far you can move a joint. Passive range of motion is how far the joint can be moved by an external force; active range of motion is how far it can be moved by its own musculature.

Reciprocal inhibition—The reflexive relaxation of a muscle not in use (antagonist) when its opposite number (agonist) is contracted.

Rehabilitation—Training to regain strength and suppleness lost to injury.

Rolfing—A school of therapeutic deep-tissue massage, with particular emphasis on connective tissue manipulation.

Ruffini ending—A proprioceptor that senses position, located in the joint.

Sarcomere—A bundle of myofibrils with a partition or disk, called a Z line, at each end. The unit of contraction in the muscle fiber. Sarcomeres and their Z lines provide the transverse striations that identify skeletal muscle.

Scar tissue—Disorganized (unrehabilitated) connective tissue.

Slow-twitch muscle fiber—"Red" muscle fiber, used primarily for endurance activities, with limited quickness. See *Fast-twitch*.

Soft tissue—As used here, muscle, tendon, ligament, and fascia: everything in the musculoskeletal system that isn't bone.

Soleus—The calf muscle next to the bone, beneath the overlying gastrocnemius.

Soreness—Pain upon use; theories abound, but no precise explanation is available for its cause. See *Stiffness*.

Specificity—The athletic doctrine that decrees that physiological changes from training are restricted to the specific systems being trained.

Spring stiffness—Resistance to stretch.

Stiffness—Loss of suppleness. Some individuals perceive musculoskeletal stiffness as resistance to movement, others perceive it as pain.

Stretching—Applying a lengthening tension.

Stretch receptor—A nerve ending that is fired by stretching.

Stretch reflex—Reflexive contraction of a muscle in response to a stretching force.

Suppleness—Lively flexibility: the ability to bend, to stretch, and to spring back easily, without injury, from deformation.

Synovial fluid—Joint lubricant.

T'ai Chi Ch'uan—A mental and physical discipline employing gentle, dancelike movements.

Tendinitis—Inflamed tendons: the most common athletic injury, whether from trauma or overuse.

Tendon—The connective tissue that connects muscle to bone.

Training—Improvement by repetition.

Underuse—Levels of use insufficient to maintain the organism's health.

Yoga—A mental and physical discipline that combines meditation with stretching and breathing exercises.

Z Line—The partitioning membrane across the muscle fiber that delineates each end of the sarcomere.

ABOUT THE AUTHOR

John Jerome is a 54-year-old writer who
covered motor racing and skiing as a journalist
for twenty years, and then fell in love with
the physiology of athletics. He has published
two books on this subject—THE SWEET
SPOT IN TIME and STAYING WITH IT—
and a multitude of magazine articles, including
feature columns in *Esquire* and *Outside*.
In the process he became a practicing athlete, competing nationally in masters swimming and otherwise investigating the limits
of athletic performance, including the
benefits of stretching. He lives in western
Massachusetts, and works at home.